KINTSUGI HEROES

Connecting Seniors:

Silver Linings – Inspiring Stories of Courage and Resilience

An anthology of senior stories.

A Companion Reader to the highly successful Podcast series.

Firsthand accounts of courage and resilience.

Copyright © 2024 by Kintsugi Heroes Ltd

All rights reserved. No part of this publication may be reproduced, distributed or transmitted in any form or by any means, including photocopying, recording or other electronic or mechanical methods, without the prior written permission of the publisher, except in the case of brief quotations embodied in critical reviews and certain other non-commercial uses permitted by copyright law.

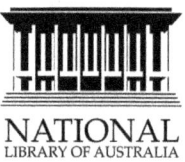

A catalogue record for this book is available from the National Library of Australia.

This book is dedicated to those people who:

Are experiencing adversity and searching for hope and inspiration.

Want to reframe their thinking to see the hidden value that adversity has brought them.

Want to learn how to better support the people around them who are experiencing life challenges.

ACKNOWLEDGEMENTS

I would like to acknowledge the following people for their contributions to this book.

NSW Department of Communities and Justice for funding the project.

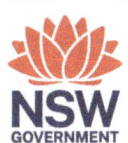

The Kintsugi Heroes who bravely shared their stories to help and inspire others:

Glenys Reid, Dr Gregory Smith OAM, Graciela Espinoza, Ian Westmoreland OAM, Don Mathewson, Jeni Vercoe, Terry James, Bradley Dowling, Narelle Gatti, Bill Kable, Jann McCall, Walter Frankel, Alex Brandt, Margaret-Anne Hayes OAM.

Project partners:

Hornsby Village Hub sponsored by the Sydney North PHN.

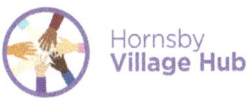

The Social Local Collective

The book production team:

John Milham – Host, Aveline Clarke – Host, Kerry Atherton – Host, Simone Allen – Host, Patty French – Author, Cecil Wilde – Editor, Kate Smith – Graphic Designer

The other members of the Kintsugi Heroes team for their commitment to our mission of:

"Helping people find their own power to heal and to be healed, by exploring their own journey and sharing it with others."

Finally, I would like to thank my wife Helen who has allowed me (albeit sometimes reluctantly!) to dedicate so much of my time, as well as our resources, into pursuing my passion projects and progressing my life purpose.

Ian Westmoreland OAM

Founder – Kintsugi Heroes

TRIGGER WARNING

Some of these stories have themes and discussion around things like trauma, isolation and suicide.

If any of these stories raise concerns with you, please reach out to someone who can support you:

Lifeline
Call: 13 11 14
Text: 0477 13 11 14
Website: lifeline.org.au

Suicide Callback Service
Call: 1300 659 467
Website: suicidecallbackservice.org.au

Beyond Blue
Call: 1300 224 636
Website: beyondblue.org.au

Mensline Australia
Call: 1300 789 978
Website: mensline.org.au

Standby Support After Suicide
Call: 1300 727 247
Website: standbysupport.com.au

CONTENTS

ABOUT KINTSUGI HEROES 11

ABOUT IAN WESTMORELAND OAM
KINTSUGI HEROES FOUNDER 12

FOREWORD BY PATRICIA FRENCH 14

    GLENYS REID 16

    GREGORY SMITH OAM 28

    GRACIELA ESPINOZA VALENZUELA 40

    DON MATHEWSON 50

    MARGARET-ANNE HAYES OAM 62

    TERRY JAMES 78

    ALEX BRANDT 90

    BRADLEY DOWLING 100

    NARELLE GATTI 110

    IAN WESTMORELAND OAM 120

    JANN MCCALL 134

    WALTER FRANKEL 148

    JENI VERCOE 162

    BILL KABLE 172

ABOUT KINTSUGI HEROES

Kintsugi is an age-old Japanese art using lacquered gold to repair broken ceramic bowls, bringing them back together as one beautiful piece.

These repaired treasures are considered more valuable and more beautiful than the original. Their gold-joined sections highlight, rather than hide, imperfection.

At Kintsugi Heroes we see this as a powerful metaphor for our own lived experiences.

In overcoming adversity, we can become stronger and more valuable to ourselves, our loved ones and our community.

The stories of the Kintsugi Heroes celebrate the scars we gather over time; the breaks, knocks and wrinkles which create their own unique beauty.

Kintsugi Heroes uses the power of storytelling to provide hope and inspiration to people experiencing life challenges.

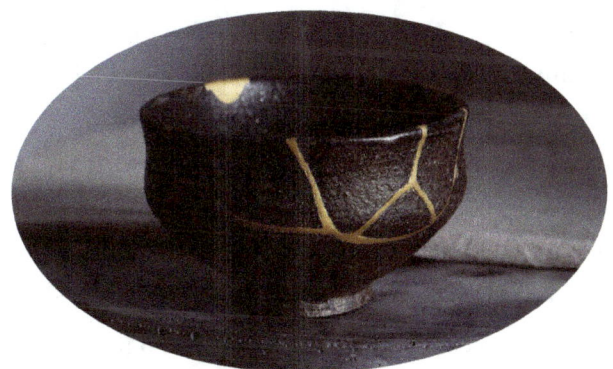

© Photo by Chris Ireland

ABOUT IAN WESTMORELAND OAM
KINTSUGI HEROES FOUNDER

Ian spent 42 years working in the Australian and New Zealand telecommunications and energy industries mainly as an IT project manager. In 2013, a profound life changing moment led him to give up paid work and commence a full-time volunteer career.

It was during his work as a volunteer for not-for-profit youth programs such as the Raise Foundation, Kidshope and COACH, Ian noticed a gap for comparable services for mature adults.

However, it wasn't until his own moment of challenge that he realised just how urgently these services were needed, especially for men, a demographic that has historically struggled with vulnerability and asking for support.

In response he developed the Mentoring Men program in June 2018, and it was officially launched as a registered charity by Julian Leeser, Federal Member for Berowra in November 2018. In just 3 years, Mentoring Men grew to become an Australia-wide, free mentoring service to support men.

With the Mentoring Men organisation now independently up and running, Ian launched another "passion project" called Kintsugi Heroes in 2022.

Complementing his previous volunteer work, Kintsugi Heroes aims to show how those major moments of challenge we face can change the course of our life, making it even more beautiful and fulfilling than ever before.

Kintsugi Heroes is a weekly podcast of inspirational interviews with people who have discovered beauty, despite the incredible adversities they have faced. It's a no-holds-barred approach that does not sugar-coat the difficult road to a life of fulfilment and hope.

Ian's story has been covered on national TV, referred to in both Federal and NSW Parliaments, and included in the best-selling Moments in Time book as well as numerous podcasts, newspapers and radio shows.

Ian and the charity organisations he established have won numerous awards including:

• NSW Volunteer of the Year award 2016 – Raise Foundation.

• NSW Volunteer of the Year award 2020 – Individual and Mentoring Men state finalist.

• AMHF Men's Health award 2020 – NSW Men's Health award.

In more recent times Ian has realised how storytelling has played such a big part in his later life, particularly as a father and grandfather.

In one of his favourite photos shown here, Ian is reading Bananas in Pyjamas to a captivated group of four of his grandkids.

Ian has been married to Helen for 41 years and they have four children and 12 grandchildren.

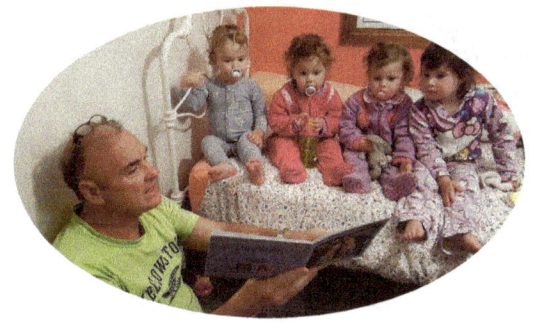

FOREWORD BY PATRICIA FRENCH

Connecting Seniors is the third book in the Kintsugi Heroes series. It tells the stories of the brave people who have come forward to share their lived experiences of adversity and how they overcame and triumphed over pain and trauma to become shining lights for others.

The Kintsugi Heroes name stems from the 'kintsugi' artform, where broken pottery is repaired with gold to create a new object with extraordinary beauty and value. We see this as a powerful metaphor for our lived experiences.

As Kintsugi Heroes founder Ian Westmoreland said, *'One of the things I talk about is finding our best life, which I define as being where we use our skills and experiences to positively impact the world around us. It is where we experience genuine contentment and fulfilment.*

'We start this life journey, heading towards our best life but then events hit us, and many are negative. We get abused, we get sick, we get influenced by social media, we have relationships break down, or we get addicted. And most importantly, we get sucked into this materialistic world and lose track of our best life. I want to encourage people to look for their best life and how they could contribute back to the community.'

The following quotes capture some of the essential values behind Kintsugi Heroes.

Mark Twain said, *'The two most important days of your life are the day you're born and the day you work out why.'*

'He was so poor, all he had was money.' Jack Kerouac (and others)

The third quote comes from Wayne Wigham, one of our Heroes, *'I'd rather have a purpose than a Porsche.'*

The Kintsugi Team arranged several community events as part of the Connecting Seniors project, including hosting a sold-out Multicultural

Dinner, where many lasting connections were made through storytelling across cultures. Another event, Our Stories Matter, featured a panel of local seniors hosted by John Milham, where wisdom and vulnerability were shared with a packed audience.

As part of the Connecting Seniors project, we also established a Community Choir. The choir includes seniors who have Parkinson's Disease and dementia or are experiencing loneliness and isolation.

Ian's dream is that every week in the local library, community centre and other venues, groups of people, maybe seniors, get together in a facilitated environment and share stories. *'This would be a great step forward to reestablish the village of my childhood full of caring and sharing. It's just waiting there to be rediscovered and unearthed again.'*

I am very honoured to be the person who takes these inspiring conversations, does a little editing and distils the essence of our Heroes' lives in their own words. In the process, I have empathised, cried, and felt anger and indignation but always resonated with the human experience before me.

As a fellow senior, I have experienced similar adversity, an inevitable part of aging. I found my solution to getting through the curve balls life throws at me is echoed by all our Senior Heroes—it's about believing that we can get through this and reframing it by having a positive attitude, self-belief, and wanting to be of service to others in any way we can.

I hope you enjoy the stories!

Patty French

GLENYS REID

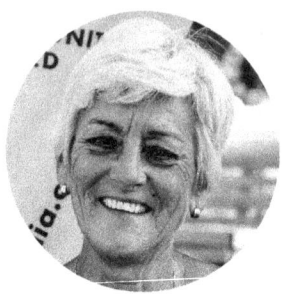

Glenys Reid is the CEO of the Chatty Cafe Foundation in Australia, an initiative focused on addressing loneliness and social isolation through facilitating conversations in coffee shops and cafes across the nation.

Glenys has a background marked by resilience, shaped by her family's experience, particularly her father's time as a prisoner of war. Her family's attitude towards life and survival has significantly influenced her approach to adversity. Glenys attributes her wisdom and values to the diverse experiences and cultures she encountered through her privileged upbringing, which included education, travel, and scholarships.

Before founding Chatty Cafe, Glenys worked in the corporate sector, facing mental health issues and employment challenges.

She places strong emphasis on the importance of physical fitness and its impact on mental health, advocating for the integration of physical activity and social connections in daily life.

She was inspired to start Chatty Cafe in 2019 after her own experiences of loneliness and social isolation led her to notice people sitting alone in cafes.

Despite various challenges, including national bushfires and the COVID-19 pandemic, she successfully launched Chatty Cafe and grew it to over 230 venues with more than 70 volunteers across Australia.

Glenys values kindness and social connection. She defines kindness as a competency and believes in the power of one person to make a difference, stressing the importance of listening to others' stories and building meaningful relationships.

I am the CEO of the Chatty Cafe Foundation. Chatty arose from my own experience of loneliness and social isolation and is focused on community members who might be feeling the same way.

When I found myself one day without a job, I felt lonely because I was used to being with a team of people, and I loved my team and job. I was quite shocked about that experience; it was unexpected and frightening.

The big moment of challenge happened for me around mid-2017. There was a period of incredible difficulty and mental health issues from 2016 to 2017, and then 2018. I was 65 and looking for jobs. I'm embarrassed to admit that when I was in a professional executive role and looked at resumés, I would cast it aside if the person was over 65. Now I was in the same situation going, oh, my God!

I'm a very skilled, capable professional with experience in government and as a not-for-profit consultant in Asia, the USA, and Australia. I spent about a year trying to get another job, and it was very difficult.

I noticed a lot of people sitting by themselves in cafes and restaurants. I'm fairly eccentric, so I would reach out and make a joke about something happening in the cafe or something else and engage that person who was sitting there by themselves.

Then, 45 minutes later, we'd be having a marvellous conversation and laughing. It was fascinating to me that those people sitting alone may be having a fine time and fully engaged in whatever they were doing, but in my experience, they were often using laptops, phones, or books as props.

They looked outwards and socially engaged with what was happening in the cafe. They might talk to the staff, but although there might be three people sitting alone at tables next to them, they wouldn't reach out. They wouldn't say, 'Do you want to join me for a coffee?' I thought it would be fantastic if people all started chatting to each other.

I had the idea to do it myself. I was going to call it Coffee Connect. A business in New South Wales had the name, so I contacted them and asked if I could steal the name from them. They said no, and then I found out about Chatty Cafe UK. They were very excited that someone might want to bring it to Australia.

That was my grand plan. I didn't have the job I used to have and still wanted, so I thought I must create one. It seemed like a good idea at the time. Little did I know what getting into a charity in Australia meant? Oh, my goodness, has that been a journey! Talk about sowing a seed, and it turns into an oak tree—I had no idea what I was getting into.

That was back in 2019, and it took off despite national bushfires. If you remember, the end of 2019 was terrible. Then, COVID-19 hit in March 2020 and went through to 2021- 22. But the Chatty Cafe is still here despite all of that.

I'm very proud to say we've got over 230 venues across Australia and over 70 volunteers who are creating opportunities through these cafes, restaurants, pubs, clubs, community centres, neighbourhood houses, libraries, etc. All of it provides opportunities for people to come together and chat. I think of it as turning lemons into lemonade. It was a serious case of lemons for me.

My family didn't take sickies or didn't cope or didn't just get on or try our hardest. That's who we were. Growing up, I developed a huge strength.

I'm aware that people face potentially similar circumstances as mine and need to seek significant help and go to clinics for help, but that never occurred to me. However, from a mental health perspective, I was suicidal, and that was difficult. I didn't go down that road, so that was the resilience in my background, and my family's attitude to life, work, and survival kicked in. Nothing like my father's experience, but I went into it saying, right, this has happened. Where do I go from here? What do I do?

For a bit of background, my father was a prisoner of war for three and a half years with the Japanese and he was in Changi and the Thai-Burma railway.

My mother was a nurse's aide in Darwin after the bombing; that was our background growing up. In that period of my father's life from 1942 to 45, he'd only been in the army six weeks when he was made a prisoner of war. He was desperate to get to the war, but it didn't have a good outcome for him. Singapore went under, and that was it.

That three and a half years defined him. Growing up, we were wrapped around that experience of him and his colleagues, the friends he made, and the friends he lost. His experiences, medically and emotionally, on the Thai-Burma railway defined him and were a key part of our life.

I adored my father. We were very similar; I am a chip off the old block. He never shared the details of his war experiences until one night when he was probably 70-something. He took a bottle of red, went into the study, and started writing a memoir. He kept a diary that he could have been killed for by the Japanese and used it as a reference tool. He ended up having the memoir published, which was great.

We were fortunate, when I look at some of the families where mainly men exhibit post-traumatic stress disorders. His friendships, which grew with the men who survived, were terribly important to his mental health. We came down every year and they marched.

He died at 88, and he marched until he was 85, despite having arthritis and other conditions. He was a very impressive man.

My mum was an amazing businesswoman before her time. She ran a company for 17 years in Canberra when women didn't run much, so I had pretty impressive parents.

My parents did not have expectations or plans for me except for the first step, when they asked me, 'What do you want to do after school?' I was unbelievably privileged and fortunate to attend a girl's grammar school, where I had an excellent education. My great-grandmother had left me some money, which I got at 21, so I could afford to go and do my physical education training in Sydney. I never forget what opportunities I had.

I went into physical education and have been very lucky from there. Many times, I was offered opportunities. That sent me to Asia on a scholarship. Then, I went to the USA on a scholarship and back to Australia.

My travel opportunities helped define me and I was exposed me to different cultures—Asia, the Americas, and all over the world. My mum loved to travel, so we travelled quite often. When I was as young as eight or nine, we went to Asia, and travel never stopped there. That exposure to different cultures gave me respect for other cultures, religions, and races.

My privileged life in Australia enabled me to continuously reinforce my good fortune and not squander those opportunities that gave me 100% in wisdom and tolerance. Time is finite; I don't waste a lot of it. Life is too exciting, and there are so many interesting people to listen to with their stories.

My experience of loneliness and separation struck home, and I learned the importance of engagement, communicating and being with people, and recognising the importance of social health. This new term distinguished between mental, physical, and social health.

It's all about the quality and importance of our relationships. It's not just about quantity but the quality of those. How it manifests itself today with me and how I express my gratitude for what has been given to me is, as much as possible, the concept of kindness, caring, and spending time with people. You're not getting caught up so much in your own schedule that you're not listening to people.

I'm a massive fan of 'Are you Okay?' Day and the switch that's made in terms of people recognising the need to reach out and ask the tough questions, having been in that space myself on a couple of occasions.

It's about kindness; that's how I try to live. It's slowed down a bit now, but we need to have time for people. If possible, we'll make time.

How would I define kindness? It's taking time to check in with people. It's a mix of being and doing. You can make food for people. That's a kind thing to do, but it's not a skill of mine, and I'm not a good cook. For me, it's more spending time with people or being in touch as much as possible. I try to take time to talk and listen to the people in my daily life and make nice gestures if I can. It might not be making a beautiful fruit loaf, but doing other nice things, giving people lifts or offering something else.

Like most things, my kindness comes from role modelling, both from childhood and life experiences demonstrated and modelled by kind people. Then, from my own personal experience, what's been most helpful when I've been in bad times, in terms of kindness and people reaching out and checking in and asking that question, 'Are you okay?'

Then, if you ask the question, you must have time to listen. You can't ask it and then move on to the next thing. It's a way of avoiding getting caught up in your own little egocentric, narcissistic world.

Always make time if it seems the right thing to do.

When things went awry in 2017, in many ways, one of the key elements of my survival was getting up and joining things. For some years, I have been part of a keep-fit group, which is called Lifestyle Adventure Training. It's been the core of me getting out of bed every morning and getting to a 06:00 a.m. class, mainly on the beach here in Hampton, with an amazing group of friends who have been part of the journey peripherally because they're part of my life, and some of them much closer.

I knew a commitment to physical fitness would significantly impact my mental health. I'm always commenting on that with the group, recognising the importance of mental health and how fitness impacts that. It's very important.

Another group meets at the same place as us, down on the beach. One of the participants in that group said to me that her group always met, and they went swimming through winter. She said, 'I always just thought it was a physical health thing until COVID came along.' She realised we all suddenly had this wakeup call that was seriously about mental health and how important it was. I love it when people get that connection. It's not just about running around, doing a few exercises, lifting a few weights, or even just swimming.

The importance of mental and physical health is profound. If we could get people out, even walking. People say, 'Can we have Chatty Cafe walking?' Absolutely, walk and chat, run and chat. I love what's happening at the moment. I'm thrilled. I don't know how Chatty can become part of it, but we've struggled to get young people on board with Chatty. The fastest growing group of lonely people is young people, 18 to 25. That's very scary.

But what's happening is they've self-generated running groups of young people. They are going for runs. I don't know what the rules are around that, but the nicest thing about it is that afterwards, they all go for coffee and have a fun social connect opportunity over a coffee. And I absolutely love that.

If we could get more young people out for a bit of a jog, have a walking group, and then go off and have a coffee afterwards, that would be sensational if it was part of a consistent lifestyle across Australia for young people.

Then people would say the cost-of-living crisis is really impacting disposable income. I'm aware some people can't afford to go to the coffee shop and have coffee.

But even if you go to your own home with a group of people and are comfortable having them come in, get yourself a Nescafe out of the jar; it won't cost you $5 to connect.

It would be fantastic if we had more of the 'pay it forward concept'. During COVID, local hospitality businesses didn't get as much acknowledgement as they should have in terms of their roles. Where I live, coffee shops have received bottles of champagne, cards, thank-you notes, and flowers. People said, 'You kept me on the planet. I had a place to come for my 1 hour out,' particularly if you're in Victoria. I came for coffee, and I met and just chatted. Even though I kept 1.5 meters distance from people on the street waiting for their coffee, I talked to another human being. That's how I maintain my mental health.

I also would like to think that cafe owners and management recognise that they have some social responsibility in terms of not just the concept of profit with purpose. Many venues that sign up for Chatty are about that. They take the money, but they also recognise that the well-being of their customers is paramount.

They're the venues where Chatty goes; if you're just in it for the profit, then that's probably not a Chatty venue. But if you're also in it for the engagement with your community and many owners, they say, 'That's what we do. We talk to the customers, and that's why we're in it. We socialise with them.'

They're sensational Chatty venues, and we don't require them to have a table or a volunteer, which some other settings do. We sip, chat, and share. The sticker just says, *'Come on in, sit down, and we'll talk to you.'* We'll encourage other people sitting by themselves, if they want to, to talk to you, too.

When I started out here, I gave no serious thought to what this meant, so I couldn't project forward. It just seemed like a really good idea. I can do that! It's been an incredible journey with a very sharp learning curve.

But we're still here and still resilient. We haven't done it perfectly because we don't have all the funding and resources, we need to do it as well as I'd like. We're pursuing those through corporate partners, grants, government, and anybody out there who wants to support Chatty. We're looking for partners and have a fantastic organisational chart regarding what we know we need and could set up. We've got people who really want to work for Chatty.

From a financial perspective, we had some brilliant volunteers. Still, at some point, you must recognise and respect that people deserve some income for the time they're putting in. That's the position I hold in that it was my decision to start it up. I don't need the funding. It would be nice to have some, but I haven't taken a salary for five years. There's nothing really to take.

But I have people who want to be national operations managers, national volunteer managers, regional managers, or state managers. People are ready to leap into those roles but we need resources to fund them.

The Chatty Cafe is vital because we live in a somewhat disconnected society. Social media, for me, is anti-social in many cases. It's counterproductive, and the loneliness statistics for young people are an indicator of that.

It's not about how many friends you have on Facebook. If you hit a rough patch, how many do you have to reach out to? Who will really be there for you? It's that disconnection element that we need to take a serious look at across Australia, which drives me forwards in terms of what we're doing.

Going into the financial year 2025, charities are doing it tough, from the biggest to the smallest. We're just a relative startup and haven't even made an annual $250,000 or anything like that.

I think the government needs to recognise the role we're playing and the need. There's real thinking around the idea that somehow, we don't need resources, people just volunteer. During COVID, one-third of volunteers disappeared across Australia, and they haven't come back in numbers, and the resources disappeared.

The separation between need and capability or capacity is getting wider. The government needs a wakeup call and the realisation that without social connection, the social fabric, and the organisation, the country will slowly diminish in its connectedness.

We're already seeing that in terms of statistics right now, whether it be crime, homelessness, suicide, or those sorts of things. A bit of money thrown our way would go a very long way to some really great organisations. We're just one initiative.

There are heaps out there. I'm not interested in competition; I'm only interested in collaborating with others to give as many people opportunities to connect as possible. That will cost them financially minimally in terms of mental, social, and physical health, and optimum outcomes.

In the future, my vision for Chatty is a combined vision across the UK and ourselves. We've got a wonderful young woman in the USA starting up Chatty in the USA.

It is the concept of chatty tables or places where customers or participants are encouraged to sit together and chat and welcome everyone at the table, no matter what the social demographic, no matter where you go, whichever cafe you walk into, wherever you're travelling and want somewhere to go and feel welcome, that's ubiquitous everywhere across Australia and that we are a welcoming country. We've always been known as a welcoming country.

We need to repair the current social fabric disconnection and then continue with the concept of mateship that we've always had in this country. Something has got lost along the way about who we are as a nation and our reaching out. We're still doing it, but not in the numbers that we need to. Reach out to your neighbours and find out who's living upstairs or next door to you.

The whole concept of multiculturalism is sensational in terms of the words we use. Still, we must work harder to reach out to people from different cultures.

But the big picture for Chatty is that we offer opportunities in social hospitality venues across Australia, whether commercial or community, whether through Chatty Cafe or anything else.

I'm a huge believer in the power of one, and nobody should underestimate their capacity, no matter what their background, to make a difference in the world. Even if it's just one person. That's where the kindness element comes in, or the bigger picture, not to get so caught up in your own stuff.

Because I'm going to do the Camino, my partner and I watched *The Way*. It's a fantastic true story about going on a trek and doing a pilgrimage about identity and finding out who you are.

I liked his comment that all the stuff and baggage we carry with us is just a burden. Get rid of all the peripheral stuff as much as you can, sensibly. I'm obviously getting older, and I'm trying to declutter. Simplify your life. Take the opportunity to think through what is important and how you might focus on it. The power of one is real, and everybody has a story. It's very much a Chatty thing.

Everybody's got a story to share, so take the time to listen.

GLENYS REID

GREGORY SMITH OAM

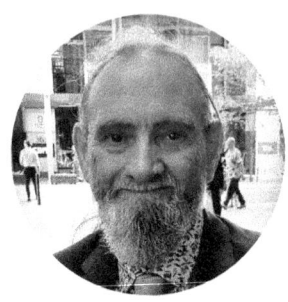

Dr Gregory P. Smith OAM is a 'Forgotten Australian' born in Tamworth, NSW in 1955. He and four of his siblings were surrendered to an orphanage in 1966. He was considered a problem child ('uncontrollable'), diagnosed as a 'sociopath' with mid-range intelligence, and was in and out of child 'care' institutions until 1974.

Following his release from 'care', Gregory searched for the skills to live a fruitful and rewarding life but became increasingly disillusioned with society and lived on the fringe as a recluse in a Northern NSW rain forest where he spent his time reflecting and reading important authors such as Douglas Adams.

In 1999, Gregory walked out of the forest and began to explore life from a different perspective. His life was transformed. In 2007 he completed a degree in Social Science, obtaining an Honours (1st Class). Gregory completed his PhD in 2015.

Today Gregory is a lecture and social researcher working to improve outcomes for the homeless and most vulnerable in Australian society. He is a Director for the End Street Sleeping Collaboration and a Special Consultant for the Global Advisory Council for CareSource USA. He is the author of the best seller Out of the Forest (2018) published by Penguin Random House, the subject of two Australian Broadcasting Corporation documentaries and a successful TEDx.

I was born into domestic violence and alcoholism. When I was two, my father picked me up by the legs and threw me against the wall, and I struck my head. That was my first serious traumatic episode, but from that point my life got worse.

I am the eldest of four siblings, and there was constant violence and anger in the house. That was my normal reality as I had no benchmark by which to measure it. This continued until I was ten when my mother gave three of my siblings and me away to an orphanage. She never explained her intent or what would happen.

I was told to jump in the car, we're going to visit an auntie in Armidale. When we pulled up at this big Gothic-looking building I saw ladies dressed in black and white. My impression was that Auntie Muriel dresses very strangely and lives in a huge house.

It turned out to be an orphanage. At ten years old, you understand who you are and the expectations around you but in those days, young people were expected to be seen and not heard. That was a very disturbing moment in my life, and set off many years of rebellion, anger, and social discontent.

After the orphanage, I became a problem child and was placed into various corrective institutions, boys' homes and reform schools. But I was never reformed and was always in trouble and would often get into fights. If I felt threatened, I would always take the initiative and move in first. As a result, between the ages of about thirteen to nineteen, I spent a lot of time in solitary confinement in concrete cells, sometimes for a week at a time with one meal a day.

Then at seventeen, I was diagnosed as a sociopath by the state psychiatrist. To put that into context, trauma wasn't really recognised at that time and it was new on the psychological and medical radar. We have our Vietnam veterans to thank for all their contributions to the understanding of trauma.

The state psychiatrist was stumped about what label to give me, so he put his hand in the hat and pulled out sociopath. So then that's who I was, a sociopath. After he explained to me what a sociopath was, I felt relieved that I knew and understood what was wrong with me.

Now I realise that all those assumptions were misaligned, and the diagnosis wasn't necessarily correct. At the time I was confused. I didn't belong to anybody and had been given away. It felt important to have a label to explain my anger and why I was always in trouble.

As I said, I was in those institutions until I was nineteen, at the 'Queen's Pleasure.' Most young people left at eighteen, but the Queen must have really liked me because she kept me there for an extra year.

A week before my nineteenth birthday, I was released and given three things, $2.25, a set of second-hand clothes and a piece of advice—don't come back.

I took the advice and bought some drinks in a pub with the money. That was my first taste of alcohol. After drinking that alcohol, I felt calm, just for a moment. It was a release of tension and a feeling I was to chase for many years.

I tried to do the right thing. But I had not been taught how to get a job, find somewhere to live or how to pay the bills. And after so much time in solitary confinement, I never learned how to communicate or be with others. I was always on the outside with emotional issues, trauma, and anger.

I tried marriage. Most men take a wife; I took a hostage. I was still angry. Fortunately, she was a little smarter than I was. So, she got out of that relationship very quickly, and all credit to her for that.

Then I wandered around trying to get jobs, the best I could do was a cleaning job or gardener, seasonal work, picking fruit. I also worked on the trawlers out of Yeppoon and did cane cutting. I always wanted to be part of society, but never had the skills.

When I was about thirty-five, I was sitting in a rainforest with the leeches all around me and the rain coming and I felt a moment of peace. When I thought about it, I felt so peaceful in that forest because people were far away, and I didn't have to be a part of it.

I could just be me, and I liked it so much that I decided to stay there for a while. During my stay in that forest, I learned a new way of surviving, and it was an adventure. I was independent and didn't have to rely on anything. Nobody told me what an idiot I was, how disgusting I was, or anything like that.

But, when I went into the forest, the problem was I took with me all that pain, trauma and hurt. I still needed to kill that pain and anaesthetise myself to a point where I could survive.

Over time, I developed ways to barter with hippies and other types of people, giving me a pretty substantial way of life. I also learned to brew my own alcohol and grow my own 'herbs' in the forest.

Now I had an unlimited supply of alcohol and herbs, and I was eating a lot of the herbs and washing them down with alcohol. That made me very sick over the years. And after five or six years, psychosis developed and I became quite ill.

After ten years I was eventually driven out of the forest because I lost an argument with some aliens.

They arrived at my campsite one evening and said, 'So you want to die in the forest?'

And I said, 'Yes.'

And they said, 'You don't want to hurt anyone else. And that's why you're living in a forest?'

I said, 'Yes, that's right.'

Then they used my own logic against me, and they said, 'Well, if you die in a forest, your body will rot, and there's a possibility nobody will ever find you.'

I said, 'Yes, that's what I want.'

And they said, 'But what about your family? What about your sisters you haven't seen for twenty-five or thirty years? You'll hurt them. They will never have closure or ever know what happened to you.'

That touched me, and I felt that at that point they had the upper hand. The deal was that if I lost that argument, I had to reconsider my position and give society another chance. I lost that argument, so, I packed my belongings in the forest and left. As I was leaving, I got hit by a car.

I ended up in hospital. I had trouble staying in the hospital. Eventually, I bargained with hospital staff because after a long time outdoors, I wasn't coping with confined spaces, so I became an outpatient.

When I walked out of the forest, I was forty-two kilos, about half the weight I am now. I needed a walking stick. I had a beard almost down to my belly button, and I probably hadn't showered for years. In the early days, I took regular baths in the creek, but the sicker I became, I bathed and washed less frequently. I suffered from psychosis, scurvy, malnutrition and the trauma as well.

One of the things that I did in the forest in the early days, is very important. I sat at the fire at night and explored my past trying to work out what had happened to me and why.

I didn't have the thoughts or the language to describe, explain, or understand what happened to me.

After a few years, I began to work it out. While it's no excuse for my father, I saw that he was like he was because he was traumatised and angry and didn't understand it. I looked back to his father and saw that cycle of abuse and trauma more deeply within my family line. I also saw the trauma in my mother's family lines, because she would agitate my father to the point of explosion.

Suddenly, it became not about blaming people but realising what had happened. I'm not saying it was appropriate, it was absolutely not appropriate to blame them. While I was in the forest, I learned that I must change things within me.

The orphanage was run by the Sisters of Mercy, who were very cruel. Admittedly, I did run away every weekend. The constabulary found me, give me a good hiding, then took me back, which also contributed to the trauma.

I knew now that I had needed to spend time away from people so that I could start to explore myself. I had given myself the gift of time to discover who I am. I needed to 'de-Catholicise.' Because up to that point, everything I did was a sin, and my guilt was heavy and an almost impossible burden to carry. I pulled that apart and looked at morality versus intent and many other philosophical concepts while I was there.

Once I left the forest, I started to regain my health through the hospital system. The social workers were brilliant because I'd forgotten who I was. They established my identity and registered me for a Disability Support Pension because I was so sick that I was expected to die within a year.

So, there I was, on the Gold Coast, in the Tweed Heads area, and with an income including three months back pay. I hadn't seen that much money for a very long time. It was very simple—what does a practising alcoholic, homeless, drug addict do with all this money?

Well, obviously, you buy a haversack and fill it up with booze and drugs. I had a cask of fruit elixir, a couple of bottles of bourbon, tobacco, marijuana, cocaine, and a little amphetamine, just in case. My priorities were only to kill the pain.

Even after everything I had faced and deconstructed, I still needed to numb the pain which had intensified because of all I had worked through. And so, in about February 2000, I was sitting on a bench behind the Tweed

Heads hospital, looking at the beautiful Tweed River with my backpack full of stuff next to me.

This was a critical moment because I thought if I only had one person that I could tell all my troubles to, I'd be okay. I felt I was the loneliest man in Australia, as my situation suddenly struck me with devastating clarity. I was forty-five years old. Everything I owned was in that backpack next to me. I had not one friend in the world.

I had a little reflection from when I was just five or six years old. I remember, it was a passion for life. I dreamed of being a fireman, a doctor, the hero, and how my passion burned at that age.

As I sat on that park bench that day, the only thing left of that fire was a tiny little ember. I just wanted to reach in and put it out. I suddenly found myself in a cloud of fog.

I became aware that I was very angry and tired, but I was ready for the next fight. All my life, I was ready for the next fight. When the fog receded, I could see my hands holding this great big double-edged sword.

I knew I was ready to wield that sword. I looked around at the devastation and destruction but couldn't see anybody to fight. I suddenly realised I'd been fighting myself all my life. There was never anyone else to fight. I tried to throw that sword away, but I couldn't.

I dropped to my knees, and thought, I don't want to do this anymore. Suddenly, I was sitting on the park bench again, and I could see the river; it was a lovely sunny day. In that moment, I decided that no matter what I had to do, I did not want to be the person sitting on that park bench.

I was willing to do whatever was necessary to change who I was, so I got up from the park bench and walked away. I left the backpack there. I've never had a drug, cigarette, or alcohol since that moment.

I thought my previous life was pretty tough, but it was about to get a lot tougher because

I was a slave to my emotions, my past, alcohol, drugs, and other people's emotions. But, I was no longer a victim. But I had to learn discernment and many other things.

I didn't have role models, so who do I want to be? Who do I want to model myself on? For better or worse, I chose a medieval knight, and what would this knight do in my situation? What would the chivalry be? What would be the morals, the ethics going forward?

I felt I needed direction and comfort in that direction. There were not many good people in the worlds I traversed. If there were, I couldn't see them because my world was so dark. So I had to turn on the lights and start shining; take the bushel off the candle.

I was still experiencing pain. Those next few years were probably the most painful of my life, but my attitude was I can take this; bring it on. I had to learn how to talk to people and accept help from people. I needed to work. I didn't want to be on the Disability Support Pension so during the first couple of years, I applied for hundreds and hundreds of jobs, but I couldn't even get an interview.

I learned that some of the skills I had were transferable to modern society. Reading signs was one of them and I can do that quite well today. I heard that computers were the way of the future, so I found a six-week free computer hardware course at Kingscliff TAFE.

I learned two valuable lessons there. Firstly, I hate computers. Secondly, I love to learn and am pretty good at learning. I decided to do my School Certificate because, in my world, that was a pinnacle of success. But I couldn't do that because TAFE's and Community Colleges didn't do it anymore. Then I learned about a tertiary preparation course at Southport TAFE in Queensland. The only word I understood was 'course.' I had no idea what tertiary or preparation were. Anyway, I got chauffeur driven up there in the Mercedes bus, and everything's beautiful.

I went up to Southport TAFE with all my arrogance and asked them to sign me up. But, they said, 'No, it doesn't quite work like that. This is a fee-paying program; you will have to pay your fees.'

I said, 'I don't have a lot of money. Can I pay it off?' And we had a chat and arranged that each Monday morning, I would come in and pay a certain amount of money. And for that week, they'd teach me. I realised my negotiation skills were improving.

It was an eight or a nine-month course. Many things happened to me during that time because I was a part of a classroom. I was a part of a group of people sitting around having lunch together and chatting. I had my first coffee ever with another human being during that time.

At that time, I was nearly forty-six. I was invited to my first-ever barbecue, while I was still sleeping down on the beach. I was still homeless. If somebody asked me where I lived, I said, quite flippantly, 'Down next to the beach. Got a nice place down there.' People didn't need to know.

I approached the counsellor at the TAFE, telling them that I really wanted to find a place to live, but I didn't know how to do it. I don't think she understood what I was trying to say because what she said to me is, 'Well, you go to a real estate agent.' I knew this, but I've never done it as I was never taught. That's the difference between mechanical skills and theory.

I'm very good at theory. It's probably one of my strengths. But when it comes to hands-on mechanical actions and processes, that's a whole different thing for me. During one my rare conversations with my sister she said, 'Gregory, you're a very intelligent man, but the problem is you have absolutely no common sense.' I took offence at that and never spoke to her for years. Today I understand what she meant, and I totally agree with her.

That TAFE course was a mind-opening exploration for me. I got through it and was even dux of the class and met the Gold Coast Mayor. I ended up with a pretty good grade point average, and I got into university. That was one of the scariest things I ever did.

I was still homeless until halfway through my undergrad. It was a long time before I was ready to transition into a sense of feeling safe because I had lived in survival mode for so long.

I had a little place on Chevron Island for a while. It was a tiny one-bedroom flat amongst all the big skyscrapers. I couldn't live there because it was so claustrophobic and horrible. I liberated a steel hub cap from a Volkswagen and collected some sticks, so I could have a little fire in the place for a bit of connection. I had a little fire every night for as long as I was there, but I had to leave. I just couldn't do it.

I did okay going through university. I studied sociology and social sciences, and this irony doesn't escape me. Towards the end, I received a phone call from one of my lecturers offering me work. I couldn't get a job; that's how I ended up in university. And now I've not quite finished my undergrad, and I'm being offered work; I'm not even looking for it.

The condition was that I continue to study. So, I did an Honours and ended up with First Class Honours, which gave me an Australian scholarship award to do a PhD which I completed in 2015. I never gave up. I was sixty-four when I received my first tenured position.

When I was sixty-seven I had the birth of my son. I work for many different companies. For example, the second largest Medivac provider in the US, basically the Medicare provider in the US, has sought me out to be a special consultant to them in specific niche areas. I've also worked on the New South Wales Premier's Priority projects to end street sleeping.

You know, life's a wonderful thing,

I've thought about the pain. There are two types of pain. There's pleasure in certain kinds of pain because there's an understanding that there will be an outcome. So, for example, the pain that kept me in the darkness ended on the park bench the day I walked away from the backpack.

The pain going forward was to bring it on, let's get this sorted. First, I needed to learn how to communicate with people. Then, I needed to learn how to be a part of society. Third, I needed to learn how to grieve and be sad and disappointed. One of the biggest lessons was what other people think about me is none of my business. And what I think of other people is my business.

Something that is important to me today is understanding pathways through trauma. And how sometimes the simplest bridges can be built to guide us through what's required, which is the willingness to be open-minded and honest with ourselves.

What I understand very clearly today is that is that there are only two things that I truly own. One is my name, the other one is my word as a human being. I own that and put that out there for other people to either trust, not trust, to accept or to judge me by, so my word is very valuable to me and what I say and what I do needs to be congruent.

Another thing I've learned is that I used to have a bad habit of interfering with my life. I had no idea what the universe had planned for me. I would always interfere, and it would always cause grief and pain. I've had to learn to put the paddle in the canoe and enjoy the view. There was always conflict and hard work. I found got very little done in a day, but if I go with the canoe and don't go against it, here's less resistance, I get more done and I'm much happier.

When I'm communicating with others or sharing stories; the stories and words are about magic. When I look up at that rear revision mirror of life and see what's behind me, all I see is treasure, no longer any pain.

There are a lot of things that fit a situation—the right shape, the right fit for a given moment.

If I'm sharing with someone, and there's something there that I can use that's beneficial to them, that's great. All I have to do is be wise enough to identify it and understand it.

Everything is exactly as it is meant to be right here. My mission, should I choose to accept it, is just merely to accept it.

What I would say to others who are going through something like I did, is to stop fighting, as painful as it is, and as scary as that is. Don't ever give up, don't put your faith in others. Trust yourself in the first instance.

I have a little gold Teddy ring here. I'd never been given a toy as a child. When I started university, I bought that Teddy bear ring because I'd identified the hurt child inside. And I realised that I needed to become a responsible parent and take care of that hurt child, so I gave that hurt child this ring

Symbolism is very important in recovery, especially a traumatic recovery from PTSD. There is also power of desire or of forgiveness, which is very important.

For me to be able to forgive my parents has freed me. It's also cut that chain on that cycle of abuse. I don't need to be like my parents, because I've understood and forgiven them. Those things that are very helpful to understand.

I now understand why I couldn't throw that double-edged sword away. A sword is not just a weapon. It's also a precious tool.

GRACIELA ESPINOZA VALENZUELA

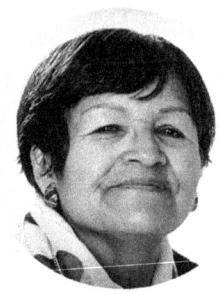

Graciela Espinoza Valenzuela was born in the mountains in Huánuco, Peru, in 1948. The second of nine siblings, her early life took her all over Peru with her schoolteacher parents. Her worldview was expanded by meeting people from all walks of life and being deeply involved with the community from a young age.

She moved to Australia with her husband of 54 years, Mario, in order to be closer to her two children, who emigrated after university. Family unity is very important to her, and in Peruvian culture.

Despite a cancer diagnosis, Graciela is involved with an offshoot of community organisation—Fusion—which aims to connect Spanish-speaking Australian migrants and help them integrate into the Australian community. There are members from 16 different Spanish-speaking countries across South America, Europe, and Africa.

My name is Graciela Espinoza Valenzuela. That is the first difference with this culture because we take two surnames—for my father, and my mother. Maybe it is long, but we are happy, and I remember my mother and father all the time.

I was born in Peru in 1948. When I was growing up my parents taught me the important values because they were both teachers.

Everybody needs to know that in Peru we have coast, mountains, and jungle. We come from the mountains. Like Machu Picchu, for example.

My department, which is like a state, was Huánuco. We grew a lot of potatoes, vegetables, very good. I am the second of nine siblings.

That is why that is another good experience for me because we left Huánuco past another mountain in Ancash. After that, we came to the capital. What is different from Australia is that in jungle, or in mountains, there is good education and discipline My parents moved to teach, so I knew different states. That is why the oldest born in Huánuco, the third and born in Ancash, and the last five siblings in Lima.

In my childhood, all the time I learned we need to overcome adversity. We needed to say, 'This is no problem. No money, no problem.' In our childhood we needed to start to organise financial problems, organise the siblings or help my parents. We socialise in the family. That is why I was growing and helping family socialise in the community. Even in Lima, in Peru. After that, here, it is the same behaviour. Because in my country, the characteristic of people is resilience. Resilience for solutions to the problems.

All the time when we learn and practiced. We do not just listen we practice the values. We start and grow the resilience little by little. Small problem solution for the small problems. After that, our brain got open and was growing, for different problems. It's like training.

It's a quality of Peru, but also Central or South America. Maybe because, Machu Picchu was the centre of all Inca Empire. But all South America, even all Spanish speaking, they similar characteristics. Different background, maybe different linguistically or maybe actions are different because each people is different. But we are happy with them because we find mostly the same things in common.

I am a person who always carries out activities in the family, in the community and social area. Because my parents were teaching me since

I was born. I studied at the St Vincent de Paul school. That is very good because we visited, for example, prison, hospital, all places or poor areas. We said because of my country or my classmates, we learn from everybody. Because the poor people teach us a lot. We learn from them too.

I studied at the university for my career as a teacher. But I couldn't work as a teacher because the salary is very little, not enough to live there. That is why I work in private companies, selling something or representing companies, brick companies, cement companies, material. Because, you know, we need to get money to give a good education to my three children. That is why they could come here.

We came to Australia for family reunion. Because in South America, especially Peru, we join with all the family. We live in an extended family with the parents, aunties, uncle, and grandparents closer. And when they came here, we miss them, Mario my husband and me. We are 54 years married. We miss the children, so we came here.

The main problem, because that is when you change the culture, you know, the first problem was the language, they never speak English in Peru. All the time, Spanish. But that is another characteristic in resilience or decision.

When we decided to do something, we do that. We decided we need to learn, maybe 100 words a week. Pronunciation, listening, writing, and reading. We decided in that form. We learn that English. And thank you so much to the church and the organisation—for example, Fusion.

Now with Kintsugi, I am learning a lot from you. Because we are practicing reading, reading all histories, reading all our news.

We needed to adapt when we came here. We needed to think it's not difficult, maybe I need to think positive things. It's not just sad. Because, you know, even in my country, if I go to another department or a state it is different. We need to adapt and equate. Here, the main problem is language. Another very hard problem, is the loneliness and isolation, because this culture is different. As I said, we live in the extended family. Here it is just basic family. It is another form of life. We need to adapt thinking and love everybody and connect.

For example, my neighbour on the right side is from Korea. The left side is from Australia. It's a different attitude, even a different form of talking. But we need to connect with everybody, because this is multicultural.

That is very good lesson for us because help of the integration of the Spanish speaking community, which was organised two years ago, we decided, we need to understand between different people, different countries. And now in a multicultural country, Australia, it is better because our knowledge is growing, that is very important.

It's not just the young people, the young, the mature people, the old people, the brain is opening, and the knowledge is growing. Our love too. Because we need to understand each other and respect and put our values in practical form. Understanding, respect, solidarity; all the values we can. That creates resilience because it's the base for the future.

When we feel sick, for example, and maybe the doctor or somebody says, 'How much are you in pain between one and ten? We think really it is five. But it's not too much. I need to think less. Because we need a contagious good attitude to the family, to the community. That is a problem too. But it's all right because we help our family, our community. We need to help give just positive things. Not to give problems, that's no good.

We have to think nothing is bad, everything is all right, or something happened for a reason. For example, if I fell down two times. The doctor explained to me about this illness. I need to look after myself. Before I didn't look after myself.

But we overcome everything with a good attitude.

You know, I am very happy. From the government, for example. The social area. Or the health area. Now it extends for everything, not just for medicine, I think that is a very good concept.

Not just medicine. In happiness. That is very good for us. But this is possible for us because when we immigrated from our countries, we brought our open mind and an open attitude to receive and learn all the good about Australia and multicultural countries. Just accept good. If we found, something looking negative, because we are not perfect, only my God, is perfect. If we find something looking negative, don't remember that. That is the best way.

What I love to do is reading and researching. Sometimes before I liked to cook food. But now I can't because of my illness. Peru mostly, and all Spanish speaking countries, has good recipes for every dishes. But now I can't do it properly. Maybe half and half.

I like traveling. By train is very good or sometimes with friends or our family. Because I like to know all Australia and I am happy when I go to a new part of each state, even Northern Territory. Two weeks ago, I was in Uluru, it was very good.

Because we need to know. All the world is similar. We have for example no Aborigines. We have indigenous people who are speaking dialects like here, in my country too. we understand these people. That is why I am very happy to know Uluru and now I have the map. How many? Maybe 200 groups all Australia, and in New South Wales too. Maybe we will have a meeting with them. With our integration of the Spanish speaking community and Australia.

When we say Australian communities, we need to think about it as multicultural. The Australian and the Aborigines too. Because these groups give lessons to us.

We are part of a Spanish speaking organisation here. Because 21 countries speak Spanish here, 19 from America. One country, Spain, from

Europe, and one from Africa, Equatorial Guinea. We already meet with people from 16 countries. We join and interchange ideas, messages, and lessons. Because each people think differently and understand differently too.

The end purpose is union for all Spanish speaking communities. For understanding.

And maybe to let this multicultural country know this is a big community. Because when we are separate, from Peru, Chile, Ecuador, or Spain, but everybody speaks Spanish.

We help all migrants when they arrive in different stages. We say to them, you need to know the law. You need to respect, you need to accept your duty and your rights, is the same level. Not only rights, because duty for us is more important. Because we need to help Australia, because the country helps us. That is the main purpose, the main objective.

That is why our passion is joining the Spanish speaking countries and integrating with Australian communities. Because they are multicultural. We connected with Singapore, Malaysia, we connect with Kenya, and they start to learn Spanish. It's, very interesting because they know our ways and that we are very welcoming. They recognise our values, but we are open to them coming without calling us and give them a cup of tea. Because we need to understand many people from different countries, maybe have loneliness too.

We need to help them, so even sing a song in English and say, 'Please, we need to sing a song,' we give them a sheet. 'Little by little you are trying. Don't worry if you don't understand. No worries.'

But you integrate, and are getting happy, getting freedom. Don't worry everybody. Or even say to them, you need to know advice for your children or your grandchildren. For example, about universities is very important. We need to advise as an organisation.

We need to advise what is better for you or for your future or for your family future. Because that is the difference. For example, in our background we worry not just for my children. We are thinking about my grandchildren. You try to do this because Australia and all the world needs to get better. Where each generation is growing and getting better.

My husband and I worked hard in Peru in different ways. Even 6:00 a.m. until 12:00 a.m. next day earning money and to give the best education. Because this is the main thing. The best education and instruction. Education is behaviour, instruction, maths, literature, everything. That is why my children came here as skilled migrants. Because we paid. They went first to United States for English. They studied in Peru, then went there.

We are not millionaires, but we prioritise our expenses. Maybe not the best pants, the best clothes. No, this is more important. Now they understand, they are happy, they said, 'Thank you. Thank you'. They used to complain they didn't have what their friends had but now it's better and they connected quickly here.

They came here one by one, mostly because I got my cancer. That is another thing, I say, 'Thank you my children,' because they supported us when we came here. They were single then, but now each has a family. I say to them they need to improve, and I need to see my grandchildren be better, that is the best help for me, that is my strength. That is my best medicine; my children understand that, and we join together. We are 12 now. Before, there were 13 in my family. One has passed, but he is here in heaven and in my heart.

We all support each other in the Spanish speaking community, we are friendly all the time. The communication is the best, with the technology now. We are learning technology too. We are going to the TAFE college for the day to learn. You know, I'm learning more than in my sixties. We see it with my family. I saw my mum last week, she is 97, and she sees me on WhatsApp and all the family by video. We communicate with everybody.

We help each other. Today, for example, a group of six Spanish community members went to Coffs Harbour by train. One of them called another member and said, 'I can't manage my mobile phone for the WhatsApp video, what can I do?'

Another person said, 'One of the six people knows technology, or has learned from the children.'

Then we said, 'You learn from your children now you teach her because when you go on a holiday, you just don't go on holiday to eat or walk, just learn something and you collaborate with the friend.' An hour ago we heard from Feliciana, 'Hello, I've learned now, I hope tomorrow I remember!'

We are all family. In our mind, the family is biological family, you know, from the same parents. But we are siblings all the world.

Yes, because we are siblings and daughter and son and children from my God. Our culture teaches this, it is a different form of love. Australians show different form. Because for example, somebody Australian, when I make a mistake, will say, 'You must say it like this...'

Thank you so much. They do not criticise; that is love too, a different form of love. Or 'Be careful or you will fall down' or asking' Are you okay?' That is a different love. We never ask like that, because we help directly. But we interchange culture and are growing culture.

I have been with my husband for 54 years, we stay connected through patience, persevering and sometimes not listening, selective hearing or say, 'Bye. I will come back. I will buy something.' We've got love.

In my culture, when we said, 'I marry in good things. I accept bad things until we pass away.' We need to do that until we pass away. It is very rare the people get another marriage in my country.

Mario and I are a team. He helps me in practical things because my body is not good now. I help him in the mind because he has started to forget a lot.

We hope to stay until we pass away together. Helping each other and forget the love, that is better.

I love to socialise, and connecting with more people, and to give us a legacy. As a legacy, the action maybe in future. Now, I am like a mentor for three people. But other people are learning, because in the future I am no longer a mentor. That is the best action. Because the people helping each other is the best. That is the main thing we need to do now. That is my goal, my passion. Joining even with another culture with family, in community and in country, maybe little by little.

We thank you Australia. We are old. My group, the six people who went Coffs Harbour for free. We say, 'Thank you Australia.' But we need to help Australia. We need to contribute a lot. We don't have money, but we need to take positive actions to get a better country. For example, now we are very worried for 12th of September. It's the local elections.

We are worried because we did not come Australia just for traveling or for dancing. We need to be responsible. Where is the candidate? What can I do?

Thinking about the local area, in Hornsby, Epping, Parramatta, each Shire Council. We're not talking about the person, or religion or politics, we're talking about, for example, health, policies, education. Politics is all right. But it is the policies that support education, support health, maybe services. We are asking what can I do with this problem?

We need to integrate. Integrating is not just joining or lying on the bed together. To integrate is thinking for the future or helping for the future of Australia. Maybe mistake. Maybe mistakes, everywhere there are mistakes. No, but we need to be thinking and say, 'I belong to Australia. I belong to Hornsby, I belong to Epping, I belong, right?' I need to be active.

We sit around and have no meeting that's too hard, just conversation. I know, maybe somebody said just vote, but no, converse. What do you think about it? What is your opinion? If you don't agree with me, I respect you. But we need to read about the rules; local, state, and federal rules. What is federal? How many councils, for example, in the state, and how many states? The capital is not a state it is a territory.

We need to learn because it's different here. We are learning about everything. We even said, 'Why are bananas very expensive now?' For example, it's for nutrition. Somebody said, 'You read what another fruit, what another dish gave you the same as bananas.' You aren't desperate to eat banana or the tomato, in that one month.'

That is financial. Because we need to help each other. But maybe we buy something, to give to somebody who doesn't have it. That is very good, it is better.

My thinking is always positive, everything in love, everything in helping each other. Or maybe if somebody doesn't smile. Look the face, but don't look just the face. Because you need to think that people are very serious inside. Maybe it is very hard for them. Like the homeless, for example. Not to criticise because maybe they didn't listen. Always be positive.

I'm sorry my English is not great.

Kintsugi Heroes is similar to our culture. Maybe, I will ask somebody, if we can talk to each (Spanish speaking) country we have people from and teach them how to overcome the adversity. The adversity is very hard all the time. Adversity in health, in help, in education, in social problems.

DON MATHEWSON

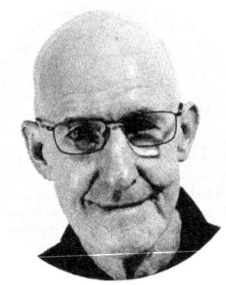

Don Mathewson is a true champion who shares his extraordinary story of courage, determination, a passion for athletics, and overcoming significant physical challenges alongside a life of service to others.

After a successful navy career, he became a field director with World Vision, then later a senior executive coach.

Don is a Masters track athlete who has been world champion on three occasions across different age groups and has received fifteen other medals. In his pursuit of excellence, he has completed World Masters Athletics Championships in Finland, the USA, France, Brazil, Spain, and Australia.

As well as holding several Australian and State records across different distances, Don cycles with an early morning group three days a week and is passionate about mature age health and fitness.

He supports others through several forms of volunteering, including Mentoring Men, teaching English as a second language, and serving on the National Committee of the Endeavour Foundation, a large disability support organisation.

I hope I'm not telling my story here under false pretensions because I don't feel like a hero, but I sometimes feel like a broken pot!

My early years growing up in Queensland were not too great. My mum died when I was twelve, and I don't have many memories of her. Then my dad remarried, but unfortunately, I didn't get on with my stepmother. On a whim, I joined the Royal Australian Navy, which at the time had a scheme where boys could join the navy between 15 and a half and 16.

This couldn't happen these days, as the UN doesn't allow young people under 18 to join the defence force. I stayed in the navy for 21 years in the navy and progressed through the ranks. I was very serious about the navy and wanted to do well.

By 24, I had passed all my exams and went to England for two and a half years of training with the Royal Navy to become a Naval Officer. After that, I served on several ships and establishments and returned to England to the Royal Military College of Science to do a Master's level course.

During my naval career, I had a profound and quite prolonged depression, which made me unfit for sea service for a couple of years. I thought my career was over, but with help and medication, I came through that, and my career reignited. I wasn't held back and was given an accelerated promotion to Lieutenant Commander, after which I served in major warships. However, after 21 years, I was still only 36 and decided to leave; one of the reasons was to create a stable home for our disabled child.

Following my time in the navy, I worked with World Vision, the international overseas aid and development organisation. I started as the NSW state manager. Then, for six years, I was the field director for the whole South Pacific region, which was fantastic fun as I travelled to villages in Papua New Guinea, Fiji, Vanuatu, and Tonga. I realised later that was where I picked up my value set of wanting to help others.

After 13 years, I joined a major human resources organisation where I was a senior manager and later a senior executive coach. I only left there recently, well beyond the average time for working.

It is essential for me to have a purpose in my life, and I loved going to work as a senior executive coach. I found that tremendously satisfying, helping people get back on their feet and uncovering who they are and what their values are. One of my favourite sayings is, 'Well, you take my advice; I'm not using it,' but I didn't give much advice. Instead, I listened and journeyed with people. Now, I volunteer as a mentor with Mentoring Men. It's tremendous doing that.

Most of the guys I've mentored are in their twenties to late thirties. I've also enjoyed teaching many of them English as a second language. I'm on an advisory group for Australia's largest disability support employer, advising the board and also meet with a young fellow in his early forties who had a stroke and is unable to speak; it's called aphasia.

But in the other part of my life, I'm an Elite Masters athlete and compete internationally. I've been pretty successful at doing that. I've been to several countries for the World Masters Athletics Championships. Every year I compete in the Australian Masters Championships. I have been the Australian Championship Champion in my age group on several occasions.

I'm a bit unusual in that I specialise in middle distance. My speciality is 1500 metres while 800 metres is probably my second best, although just a bit short for me and I've never won that event. Another good event is the 5000 metres, but I've never won the world championships, although I won many times elsewhere. I also run ten kilometres on the track. The world championships last ten days, and I run the half marathon on the last day.

The adversity that I really want to talk about is regarding my athletics. Which on reflection has been more serious than I've given it credit for.

I've always been a runner. I've done many cities to surfs and won three trophies for city to surf in my age group. When I met a man who is now my coach, he suggested I train for the track. Then I realised that I'm a middle-distance runner.

I competed at my first World Masters Athletics Championships in Finland in 2009. I was very excited but didn't know the competition or what was ahead of me. But eight weeks before the event, I did a hamstring injury which derailed me. Still, I got over it and won the 1500 metres world and came second in the 800 metres, and we'd already won the cross-country team goal medal, which was the first event over the ten days. That was my first introduction, and it was a pleasant surprise.

The next world championships were in Sacramento in 2011. I had an online Olympic coach I had never met, but he kept me honest. I thought I would do very well, but I was beaten and came in third place to well-known American and Spanish guys.

I came second in the 800 metres, and I've raced that guy several times since and been world number one. Every year you get a world ranking on several occasions in my age group, and things went bad in the lead-up to it. After that, I was running well, just the occasional injury you get over with massage and stretching.

Then, three months before the 2013 World Championships in Brazil, I was doing some push-ups. It was the middle of winter and freezing, and I did too many. When I got into bed my head started pounding with terrible pain. This wasn't normal; I was groaning and screaming when the ambulance men came. I didn't know it then, but I'd had a brain haemorrhage.

Most people die before they get to the hospital with a brain haemorrhage, depending on how bad it is. As soon as I got in the ambulance, they gave me some great painkillers, and within fifteen minutes, I was feeling really good and chatting.

My neurosurgeon in the ICU was an ex-naval surgeon. We got on really well, and he said, 'Look, Don, we've done every scan we can, but we can't find the source of the bleeding. This could mean you could die any second while I'm talking to you, or you're going to be okay.'

After seven weeks of walking in pain, I met him, and he said, 'You can now return to your normal life. We've done many scans, and you can train as hard as you like. You're not in danger of having another brain haemorrhage, there's nothing wrong.'

I was nervous, but I trained as hard as I could seven weeks before the event. He warned me not to have high expectations and said, 'You had a major and serious illness, it's taken it out of you, but you can run.' I did run and came seventh in the 5,000 metres; but people were lapping me, which was very embarrassing.

I did the 10,000 metres and wrote and told him how I'd gone, and he was amazed and happy. When I was in Brazil at the start lines, my coach and friends said, 'You are on the starting line, and that's a major achievement; you are here with us.'

I learned from that experience that I didn't have to win. I wanted to win but couldn't; it was just impossible.

When I started training again, I was afraid because I had a friend who'd had a similar sub-arachnoid brain haemorrhage. It wasn't a stroke; he just burst a blood vessel, but he had a bad time and took months to get back.

However, I was back into running after seven weeks. The coach pushed me, but I was a bit afraid to go fast. My friends were very supportive, so Brazil was a learning for me.

I also cycle and one year later, in 2014 I was flying with a group in a Peloton. But the guy in front of me stopped more or less suddenly. I missed him, but the man behind me hit me. I hit the ground at 30Ks and was in a lot of pain, but didn't know what was wrong.

I went to ICU again, and the intern doctor said, 'You need a hip replacement. Your pelvis is broken in two places, and you've broken a couple of ribs.' I did not react well as I was in so much pain and gave this young doctor a bit of a serve. She said, 'I'm going to have to talk to the boss about you.' The boss was the orthopaedic surgeon.

I lucked out again with a fantastic orthopaedic surgeon, just like my neurosurgeon. He said, 'No surgery is needed. There is a bit of a lip there, but you keep running; just take three months off.'

The orthopaedic surgeon encouraged me and introduced me to a trainer. He said to him, 'This guy's a world champion runner, he is going to be back to running, and he'll never get arthritis in that spot.' That's never been a problem for me.

I took three months off and came back slowly with exercises and exercise physiology, which I took very seriously as I don't do things in half measure. When I went to the exercise physiologist, I did everything he wanted me to do.

The next event was 2015 and the World Masters Athletics Championships in Lyon, France, where I was going to have my big comeback. In 2015, I won my speciality event, the 1500 metres, by quite a long way. I was third in the 800 metres.

The next world championships were in Perth, Australia, the following year, 2016. Unfortunately, at the end of 2015, I was diagnosed with prostate cancer and was told I needed surgery.

But my doctor said, 'We're not going to do it until after the world championships in Perth; we'll fall in with you.' He was not giving me advice but enabling me to do what he obviously felt was more serious for me.

I went to Perth, and while I'm not really a cross-country runner, I won the world cross-country. And I was so cock-a-hoop, and when I was interviewed on Channel Seven in Perth, they asked me if I did this for social reasons.

I said, 'No, it's not. I come here for one reason, I'm here to win.' I realised that I was saying things that weren't very humble, so I added, 'But the social life is very important to me as well.' I got myself out of it. It was on TV that night, and I didn't see it, but I'm still embarrassed about it.

Then I came back and had my surgery which meant more time out. But it didn't worry me; my surgeon is a runner, so he understands me. That was another very positive event for me.

I hadn't paid much attention to that cancer in 2016, but in 2021, I had excruciating pain in my lower back and couldn't walk. I thought this was it; my running days were over.

I was already being treated for arthritis in my lower back when an MRI showed a growth on the nerve roots in my lower back.

After being told by other doctors that I couldn't see my preferred neurosurgeon, I sent him my MRI and quickly got an appointment.

He showed me the damage to my nerve roots and the nerves and said, 'Your nerves are not working.' Then he asked me a few questions, resulting in urgent surgery the same week. A large benign growth that had been there for a long time was removed. The following day, I got up and walked around the corridors pain-free after eight months of pain.

That was probably the worst experience, but it all happened quite quickly. The next day the surgeon came in and after an examination, said I could go home today. I would eventually be able to get back to running but needed to take it easy.

I have made a slow and painful comeback and easily won my five events at the Australian Championship in March this year.

My physician friend, a well-known runner, told me they call me the 'man of steel' because whatever happens to me, I get over it and always come back.

When I think about the hardest thing for me to deal with throughout the pain and these events, it wasn't the pain. That was terrible, but I overcame it and was lucky to have the medical advice I got from people who understood me and knew what my drivers were.

I'm strongly motivated. A friend gave me feedback I'd never thought about before. He told me people say I am very competitive, but I didn't realise that.

Another friend told me there are two things about me. One is that I am very competitive, and that's a good thing. But there's a bad thing about me; I am very competitive, and my competitiveness can be like a two-edged sword. I'm glad I'm competitive, but that wouldn't be a value I would put out there. I would never say that, but I've had to face the truth that I am competitive and want to win. My competitiveness has helped me get through the physical and emotional setbacks I have experienced throughout my life.

Many of my younger friends are outstanding athletes. One of them is an iron man, and he's also one of my coaches. I run with a group of young triathlon trainees, including some girls, from 10 up to 16, and I train with them, and I do well. There were one or two older people, but not many.

My coach is so positive to me. When I'm running, they say, look, there's a world champion. That's a competitive guy; look at him. I never mention my age.

A couple of weeks ago, we were at the world championships in Perth, where I was running the cross country. We were chatting with the young ones; seven of them had qualified for the Australian Cross Country Championships in Adelaide, and they were going, it's a big deal.

And Shannon, the coach, said, 'You've got to have the mindset to win;

I didn't have the mindset to win.'

I said, 'You know, I was in that world championships too? And I won in my age group; I knew I would win from the beginning because it was a flat course.'

That sparked a fantastic response from all those young guys high fiving me; it was wonderful. This might not sound too humble, I didn't aim for that response, but they felt inspired by having me there.

I'm not there for that reason. I'm there for me. It's lovely and joyful for me to run with those young guys every week. But for that coach, to have me there, it's an inspiration.

What has helped me as well is that I believe in myself. I have an attitude—I don't dwell on this—but my attitude is that I can get through this. It's not good now, but through the process and from experience, I know that life is hard. You don't know what's around the corner.

One of my significant learnings is that although I can sometimes feel like Superman, I am not Superman. Things can happen, they can happen to me tomorrow. I don't want to think it's going to happen. At some deeper level, maybe I overtrain. I know I can overdo it, but it's about having that mental attitude that life is fragile.

You don't know what's ahead, so have a more positive mindset. I think you know my story about ageing. I have many friends who are older than me, and some are my age who appear older. Because they often say, 'Look, oh, I'm getting old. What's that guy's name? What's that person's name?'

If people say, 'Do you mind if I ask you how old you are?' I reply, 'I never tell people my age. But, if you want to hear my philosophy of ageing, I will tell you how old I am.'

Don't focus on your age; just live life for the moment; the sun is shining, your running, your friendships, the coffee, and what's important.

Once, I ran a 10K race on the Gold Coast with two much younger women. One was in her twenties, and she said, 'Oh, you're running so well.'

Although I thought that was a bit patronising, I said, 'Okay, thank you.'

Another younger woman who I passed during the race came up to me and said, 'You're running so well. Can I ask you how old you are?'

I replied, 'It was my birthday yesterday, (a bit of a lie), I'm 70.'

She said, 'I hope I'm going to run like you when I'm your age.'

At the end of the race, she was embarrassed and said, 'I'm so sorry. I didn't mean to say that.'

I said, 'That's all right.'

Whenever I say that to anybody, my wife disappears from wherever we are, but it's a mental attitude. I realise I'm fragile, and things can happen, but I don't want to dwell on it too much.

In my dark days of injury, the depression comes out. I feel that life is hopeless, and I'll never be able to do it again. But I've learned that those times pass as the depression passes. Usually, I'm a very good human. I don't tell jokes, but I try to make light of things.

I never thought I was inspiring anybody; it's just the joy I get from being there and competing. What's essential for me, in terms of my own mental health and satisfaction, is having a purposeful life.

My athletics, cycling and teaching English to beautiful people, doing the things I do, and my mentoring are purposeful. I know I could do more, but they give me that sense of purpose and a value set around helping others.

Even as a naval officer, one of my captains said, 'Lieutenant Matthewson, you are a serious young officer.'

I didn't know what that meant then, but I am a serious person, despite the humour, who gets the best from his men. That's a long time ago, and it was because of how I handled the people I was responsible for.

I think that's what comes through, that sense of helping others. But I don't ever say helping others. My language is journeying with others through their life journey and trying to uncover wholeness for people, including myself.

When I finish a mentoring session, I feel good. I don't do advice but anything I do say, hopefully, I demonstrate. But I will say this to anyone who needs to hear it.

It's having that sense of 'you can do it.' You can overcome what's holding you back; sometimes, it takes effort. Don't be lazy because overcoming any or all those injuries takes discipline.

I am a disciplined person, including around diet and reading. I read a lot, and I read a lot about mature age health. I'm also into social justice, strongly aligned with many things, which I also read about.

My life is about having purpose and trying to see beyond what's holding you back now.

I believe exercise is vital for your mental health; you can exercise starting slowly. With our coach and training team, we have people who could be anybody, starting from the beginning, obese, or never run before. You could come and join us because we're inclusive and want you there.

We have people with deep depression in our running group. Because I've experienced that, I know the pain that people experience, and that helps me come alongside people.

Become involved in something that's community oriented. Walk in the morning in the beautiful sunshine if you can, in nature. I do that a lot; I'm not always running.

Find friends. Research shows very few people have more than one or two friends or even one with whom they can share all their innermost thoughts. I have that person, he's much older than me, and I call him my mentor. He doesn't understand what I'm talking about but listens to me.

Look for someone who listens to you but who will not give you advice. I don't want anybody to give me advice. I want someone who'll listen and say, 'Well, gee, that must have been hard, or that's tough; how are you going? Are you okay?'

MARGARET-ANNE HAYES OAM

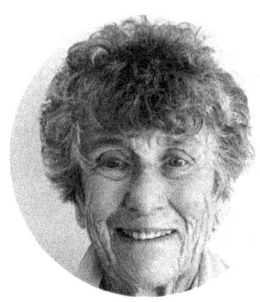

Margaret-Anne grew up in post-war Australia, experiencing a tough childhood marked by community support and church, yet overshadowed by her father's unresolved trauma.

She learned her values from her mother including the importance of empathy, kindness and helping those in need.

During the severe drought of 1994, she launched a grassroots drought appeal, mobilising her community to collect and deliver essential goods to affected areas. A lifelong commitment to fundraising and community service followed, starting locally then expanding to larger initiatives like cancer research.

Despite personal hardships, including losing her son Aaron to cancer, she remained dedicated to her community work.

She organised vital relief efforts for victims of the Cobargo bushfires, using social media despite limited technical skills. Margaret-Anne participated in skydives and shaved her head multiple times, raising substantial funds and awareness for various causes.

Her unparalleled community service earned her an Order of Australia Medal (OAM).

'What I'm most proud of is saving another mother from losing her son from a physical cancer. Whereas I lost my son to a cancer of the soul, a cancer of

the heart. I lost my son to grief… and that somewhere in that $250,000, or, as the actuary says, half a million, is the means whereby this other mother of my age still has her son.'

My journey started in 1994 when I was about 54, and there was a severe drought everywhere. I used to wake up at 18 minutes past five in the morning and walk or jog around Kokoda Avenue at the bottom of a hill.

I don't have any psychic powers, but as I was coming down the hill back home, a voice said in my head said to me, 'You need to start a drought appeal scheme', which I thought was a bit weird.

I called the scheme Women of the North Shore to Women of the Northwest, but it was basically me. This was well before computers and mobile phones. I had an electric typewriter, and I typed on two pages, double-sided. It started off with questions like, 'Have you had a cup of tea today? Have you had a hot shower?'

I printed it at home and started handing it out in the streets around Kokoda Avenue. It must have been like a seed dropped in warm soil because it took off. Over the next 18 months, wonderful donations and people came to help me pack up. It got onto the radio and into the papers.

We lived up a very steep slope and there were steps into the house and inside the house, so I would have been the fittest 54-year-old in Australia, carrying all these boxes of the most unbelievable stuff.

I realised I needed somebody to take it around. I'd never done anything like this before. I put the word out, and a couple came with a truck. We gradually took stuff all over New South Wales, going to Cobar and all those faraway places.

I didn't know then what I know now. It was September, so I started packing Christmas cakes, Christmas puddings, and other stuff and toys. I should have sent all the things to various areas so that it could all be sorted out.

When I did the bushfire appeal in Cobargo four years ago, we did the same thing. We packed everything in boxes and sent it to Cobargo. Previously, I was trying to pack everything that was needed. Basic things like tea, coffee, sugar, toilet paper, and hand creams, and all these things kept coming, as did beautiful clothes.

I did that for about 18 months. I used to pack these heavy boxes, small and large, pick them up and carry them downstairs to the truck.

It was more than 40 degrees, over 100 degrees Fahrenheit, and I thought, how on Earth did I get all those boxes down these stairs on a slope? Then I brought 33 women down to Sydney for a weekend. Local people boarded them, and we took them to the Intercontinental Hotel and cafes and to breakfast at Mrs Macquarie's Chair. I had a whole church hall full of clothes for them.

A coach came from nowhere, brought all these women down, and took them back again. We had the most unbelievable time.

I don't remember how I connected with them. There were phone calls, and I talked to everybody. I was in the local paper; it was before social media. We sent $100,000 worth of goods—everything you could think of. Not the kitchen sink, but for some reason, for there and for Cobargo, we sent up a laundry sink.

We sent many Christmas presents for children and adults. When you think back, it was amazing.

What also drove me to do that was that each night when I go to bed, I have a snugly warm bed or, if it's summer, a nice, cool bed. I've had a shower, clean clothes, and food in my tummy. I usually give thanks that there's no knock on the door at 3 a.m. when the Nazis came to take my Jewish forebears away, or I'm not in whatever disasters are happening at the moment.

I've collected beauty all my life, so I've got a house filled with beauty, 90% of it bought from op shops, markets, or fairs, but a house filled with paintings and pottery, glass, books and carpets, beautiful bone china and mugs.

Every time I see somebody's house burnt down, I see in some people the strength of saying, 'They're only material goods; we're all alive.' I think you must be the bravest people I know. Because to lose everything in my house that I've collected for, well, not for 84 years, but certainly for over 60 years now, would break my heart. Because I would miss it, and so much beauty would have been destroyed.

With the bushfires, I thought about what it must be like to lose everything, your photos, and for people older than me to lose their houses. Many of the people down in Cobargo were women in their late sixties, seventies, and eighties. They'd gone down there 40 or 50 years ago and hand-built their houses. They had no superannuation or insurance, and suddenly, at my age, they were homeless.

This time, we did have social media. I got on the phone and rang the nearest big town to Cobargo, saying, 'Can you put me onto somebody in Cobargo? I'd like to send some stuff down for the bushfires.' They gave me the name of this wonderful woman, Chris Walters. I said, 'Hi, Chris. My name's Margaret-Anne. I'd like to send you some stuff for the bushfires. What do you need?'

She said, 'Well, people have lost everything.' When they'd all been evacuated to the showground, she and another wonderful lassie decided to take over, and they started the Cobargo bushfire relief centre days after the fire. That finished about two months ago.

All I can think of is 41,000 people in Gaza, two-thirds of them being women and children, being murdered by Netanyahu, who's obviously channelling Hitler, and now Lebanon as well.

I put myself in the women's place, thinking, what must it be like to have to buy water? What must it be like to be unable to put the washing machine on and clean your clothes, get up in the morning and turn on a tap for a cup of tea, or know you've got enough money to feed the children?

It started for me with my mother. She worked in a factory or retail, and my father was a plumber. Down the street were people with big families who were always in trouble. Mum always helped. I've been given a sympathetic nature or something, but I always find myself doing what John, the minister of Wayside Chapel, says not to do.

I was born in 1940, so when I was ten, people were still recovering from the war and coming back from the war. The men were having nightmares. There was a lot of domestic violence because they didn't know what was happening. There was very little help for them. There were no building materials. We lived in a rented house. Not everybody had cars; we didn't always have a car. My father had greyhounds, so a couple of times, we had cars.

Everybody was poorer than today. There were always the rich, but they weren't the mega-rich. Of course, everybody went to church. My mother and father didn't, but I went to Sunday school, and everybody went to church, and Billy Graham was around then. There were always the crooks and the madams, but they were in King's Cross. They weren't ordinary people.

But my childhood was one of total and utter fear. My earliest memory was my father kicking to pieces my doll set when I was very young. I spent the first 20 years of my life with my stomach curling in fear if I went home when my father was home before me, and I could smell his smoke.

The kids next door, Kenny and Jim Webb, they'd run down the street to their father. They'd see their father coming; he would open their arms and swing them around. I'd see my father coming, I'd run in, and I'd be wetting my knickers, and I'd say to my mother, 'Daddy's coming, Daddy's coming'. Despite all this, Mum still helped everybody until she left.

But I don't know that anybody helped us, to be honest.

It wasn't physically violent. It was my father going through his own grief. He was obviously very clever and got a scholarship to Christ's Hospital, a school built in the 1400s in England. But then the family couldn't afford uniforms. A couple of years later, the old boys paid for the scholarship boys.

He went as a cabin boy on a ship when he was about 13 or 14 and suffered physical, practical, psychological and sexual abuse.

I think he used his own grief, which he mitigated by drinking a bottle of sweet sherry. Yet, he was brilliant and trained all those who went on to be plumbing engineers or have businesses. My mother left when I was older because she couldn't cope anymore. I don't know why; I have no idea.

I always find myself trying to help people by giving them a call or dropping around with a cake. I've always done it. I don't know where it comes from. Even now, particularly the last terrible 18 months of coping with Wayne's living nightmare in the nursing home, I've done it.

Even now, I have a few friends going through some tough times, and I like to call or text them. I think with the homelessness, with domestic violence, and the world situation, there's a need for kindness.

There's a need for love and a need for a lack of nastiness. I'm on the ABC book review now, but even there, people write nasty comments.

All through COVID, I put a joke every day on the Turramurra-Wahroonga Facebook page for four months. Most of them were terrible jokes, but, even now, somebody says, 'You and a friend got me through COVID; I used to think, if Margaret Anne's joke's there today, I can survive another day.' People keep saying this to me.

I'm technically incompetent, but I was putting these funny little things every day because I said, 'We need to have something each day that gives us a lift or takes us away from the turmoil of the world.' Since COVID, I think we've lost a lot of love, kindness, patience, and understanding.

I'm as bad as anybody. I won't tell you what happens when people cut in front of me in the car. I am considering meeting some sailors to see if they know any more language I could use. I only know about two really bad words, but I use those quite proficiently in the car until I forget somebody is with me.

I finished reading a book last night, which has really affected me and made me think that the way to start looking at life now is when you wake up in the morning and think that today's the first day of the rest of my life. How am I going to bring a bit of joy into the world? How am I going to be kind? How am I not going to whinge all bloody day? How am I going to find some inner patience and love?

Joy is incredibly hard at the moment. I've known my husband, Wayne, for 54 years. He's in hospital, in an aged care home with late-stage dementia, Alzheimer's. The people upstairs from where he is lie in a bed all day. He's had it for about ten years, and it is overwhelming.

What is interesting is the difference between those who understand and those who don't. We used to see a lot of our lovely next-door neighbours; now, we barely see them unless I go in there. He keeps saying, 'I feel awful. I haven't been to see Wayne,' yet he doesn't go and see Wayne.

Wayne's only had one or two people go to visit him. Perhaps I expect too much from society or friends, but this afternoon, somebody's coming around, I got an email. I sent an email out with pictures of Wayne looking as he is now, saying how tough it is with Alzheimer's and what a journey it is.

Sometimes, I feel incredibly angry. I tried to save Mum from Dad for the first 20 years of my life, and now, for the last 10 years, I've been looking after Wayne, and yet he's looked after me all my life. Since I lost my son, Aaron, my life changed. He was 42, and four months, and 28 days old.

I spent ten years or more and raised $250,000, but I've raised a lot more on a second level because $150,000 of it was used on 15 occasions; $10,000 was used for seed money, including cancer research.

We've now raised $33 million. It was all started by one woman, Annie Crawford. I started off with one of my dearest friends, who subsequently died. I said, 'Darling, if you don't die, I'll lose 20 kilos, and we'll both go in Annie's ten thousand.'

Well, I lost the 20 kilos and did the 10K run. I've written a story about the first night of the training, the coldest July night in 32 years. You couldn't see the end of the other side of the oval. They said, 'We'll run three times round the oval to warm up.' I thought, that's me finished. Then, I did a half marathon the next year and won. We used to listen to these wonderful researchers who came and gave us talks on a Wednesday night. We used to train on Wednesday night and Saturday morning.

I became obsessed with raising the money because I couldn't save Aaron from dying. I thought, I'm bloody sure I'm going to save another son from dying.

That's been my criteria. I couldn't save my son Aaron. But I know what I see. This woman is my age now, and she has a 62-year-old son. He's married, and she's got grandchildren; she's so happy.

The girl who started Can Too, who's raised 33 million, has lost her beloved sister, who I've also known since she was 19. A rare bile duct cancer. She said, 'I've raised all that money and couldn't save Georgie.'

An actuary said I've most likely raised well over half a million dollars from my money and the seed money. I hope that's made a difference because, otherwise, what would have made a difference?

Whatever you give out, you get back a million-fold. Those wonderful, beautiful people in Cobargo have become my friends and enriched my life. You don't realise how much you get given back. What do all those wealthy people with billions do with their money?

We raise money and support people. People came from everywhere for Cobargo. We took down 17 loads of the most wonderful things, everything anybody could wish for, except a new house. Somebody rang and said, 'I need an air conditioner.'

I said, 'I'll get you an air conditioner.' I thought, where am I going to get an air conditioner from? Anyway, I got an air conditioner and sent it down. The family that got it lost their farm and their house. They managed to convert a shed, and she had cancer. Because of the fires, you couldn't go and have the treatment.

A friend who makes $500 to $1,000 jumpers sent down three boxes. $10,000 worth of clothes. That lady got the air conditioner and those jumpers.

One night at 7:00 pm, I got a phone call from a guy named John. He said, 'Margaret-Anne, it's minus three outside, and we're as warm as toast in here with our air conditioner, and my wife is wearing one of Jane's beautiful jumpers.'

Then you think, 'It was worth it all, just for that.'

The kindness of people here, the things they donated. This February, we did Cuppa for Cobargo at the South Turramurra Uniting Church and raised another $5,000.

Then, I got an OAM. It's quite funny. A couple of days ago, I got an email from a lovely friend in England. She said, 'Didn't you get some sort of an award?' I said I got an OAM. There were 552 awarded on Australia Day.

People wrote lovely things about me, and I got some beautiful congratulations saying how much I deserved it and all that. I don't know whether that's true or not, whether I did deserve it. The saddest thing is that apparently it was put in about four and a half years or so ago and then the paperwork was lost, so after all the help he gave, Wayne couldn't understand or come to Government House.

But the people at Government House knew that he was poorly, and they made a special announcement for him when they called me up, which was lovely.

I met David and Linda Hurley, the governors-general, as I call them. I'm a little girl with no background or education, and there I was, sitting next to David at Government House dinner. They came to a couple of my fundraisers, so I was on first-name terms with the governors-general, and what a joy they were.

The second time I did a skydive in Richmond, David was the first person to give me a hug. The reason I did that was I thought if you're sitting across the desk from an oncologist who says to you, 'You've got cancer,' the fear must be insurmountable.

I'm terrified of snakes and heights, so not even for Can Too could I touch a snake.

Instead, I did two skydives. They each raised about $15,000. The first time was with a gorgeous. 40-year-old Italian ex-paratrooper. As I say to the ladies, you get very close to your skydiving partner. God help us if you have any breaking wind! I wore beautiful Joy perfume and was dressed in this great ugly tracksuit. I was still quite fat then, and it was terrifying.

The first terrifying bit was when the pilot came over and said we're 3000ft above sea level. I thought, 3000ft, we've got another 11,000ft to go, I'm going to die. What saved me was a young kid of about 25 who went grey. I was trying to say to him, 'Are you all right, pet? Are you alright?'

I was the third person. The next terrifying thing is when the shutter door opens, and suddenly, zoom. We're sitting there, and it goes off, and you jump off. It is so terrifying that I cannot tell you. Well, I can; it would be like touching a snake.

But last year, I thought, perhaps I could touch a snake and raise an extra quarter of a million dollars. Then Wayne got sick, and the sad thing is that I don't know how long this journey with Wayne will take. It exhausts me every day, so I can't take on doing a big fundraiser, which would take me eight months to organise. I'm doing the flea market at the Uniting Church. In two weeks, we raise $37,000, which goes into the community, so I can do things on a small level.

I've shaved my head for fundraising a few times, and I was awarded local woman of the year for two years. Now they make this enormous fuss, but I remember Barry O'Farrell saying, 'Oh, you're the local woman of the year.' I think I did go into Parliament House, but there was no fuss made or anything.

One of the things I also did was I saw something in the paper about the poorest town in New South Wales was a place called Gwabegar. Once again, I rang information asked for a number for anybody in Gwabegar.

I spoke to somebody in Rotary and said, 'I believe you're struggling.' When the newspaper announcement came out, they had lost their CWA Hall. I said, 'I'd like to send some stuff up. Once again, I collected masses and masses and masses of stuff, and somebody, once again, I found a truck, and we took it all up to Gwabegar.

Although I've been lauded with accolades, the other day, I went to Bendigo Bank, which has now moved to Linfield from Turramurra. I thought about how my parameters had changed. Here I am getting very excited, going to morning tea at Linfield at the Bendigo Bank, but it was lovely.

Michelle, the branch manager, and Sharon, the community manager, were there, and they gave me a hug. Another lass came out, Tracey, who said, 'you helped us with The Men's Kitchen.'

I said, 'Oh, God, did I?'

She introduced me to a friend and said, 'Margaret-Anne is a mover and a shaker. She's an icon in the community.'

'I said, 'For goodness sake, don't believe a word she says.' We chatted about the flea market. They're all volunteers, so they make up hampers to sell and raise funds, and that's all volunteers.

As I went out, there was a lass I couldn't remember, about my age, with her daughter who said, 'You look so lovely, what a beautiful dress.'

Her mother said, 'Margaret-Anne always looks beautiful; she's a pillar of our community.'

Driving home, I thought to myself, 'Isn't that lovely?' I told my daughter Abigail on the phone, 'Something lovely has happened; it lifted my spirits.' I told my son, 'I'm going to boast a bit.' This is what happened and what these people said.

He said something like, 'A prophet is without honour in his own country, on his land.'

It was lovely at Government House. I thought they were never going to stop talking because they read out what you've done. Somebody said to me, 'It was so lovely to meet you because yours was a genuine OAM.' The lovely chap next to me had been in the wine business for 40 years, but mine was as a volunteer.

It's really for the ladies who work at Fusion or the op shops; when you walk in, say, 'Hello, darling,' or 'How are you, dear? Can I help?'

I've always written. Every night when I go to bed, I write letters, articles, or begging letters. That's my trick for fundraisers. You always go to the top, go to the chairman or the CEO. I'm lucky because now I can start off dear so and so. I bet this is the first letter you've received from an 84-year-old skydiver. Hopefully, that gets them in.

What I'm most proud of is saving another mother from losing her son from a physical cancer. Whereas I lost my son to a cancer of the soul, a cancer of the heart. I lost my son to grief. And what I'm most proud of is that somewhere in that $250,000, or, as the actuary says, half a million, is the means whereby this other mother of my age still has her son. That's what I'm most proud of.

What I want to pass on to people are the words *'be kind'*. The other thing is to try to not be like me and be filled with guilt. I cannot stop thinking I'm the most selfish person I know.

But be kind. If you see somebody who needs a hand sometimes, all it needs is the touch of a hand, a phone call, or, if you have to, some bloody texts. You don't have to make casseroles, or soup, or anything I've done all my life.

I see beauty in this world. Now, I'm looking at a beautiful pink rhododendron. There's beauty in people's faces and in people's souls. I think perhaps you should have a bit of patience with yourself. Try to see that whatever you've done, you've most likely done the best you can.

See the joy in the world and like that funny old meme—dance; if nobody's watching, get out there and dance. That's what I've decided. I will start and put some rock and roll on every day to dance to and sing. I've got a voice like a crow, but during COVID, I used to do these funny things of myself, singing Zippity Doo Dah or What a Beautiful Day, dressed up in long gowns, and people loved them.

Most people want essentially a warm bed, some food in their tummy. They want to know their children are safe. For young people these days, with that twelve-year-old girl suiciding for bullying; it all goes back, doesn't it, to being kind?

My earliest memory at church was, 'Do unto others as you would have others do unto you.' I always used the King James version of the Bible.

It's reasonable if you put yourself in their place, or if you think I'm in that place now, what would they do for me? President Kennedy said, 'Not what your country can do for you, but what you can do for your country.'

You don't want to do it as far as your country. You should do it for your neighbour or a friend you haven't talked to. If I get friends in my mind, I've got to ring them. I'd like to believe, as Shakespeare said, 'There's more in heaven and earth than this world dreams of.' I think, in a way, there is.

I don't have any of those skills, but I have one or two friends who do. So, be kind and be as patient as you can. It's not always possible, especially with these bastards that drive before you, but try to understand it. It doesn't matter if. If you're in Gaza or if you're in Israel, Lebanon, or America, you want what is best for those who love you.

If anybody's around who's wealthy, you don't need ten houses. When people were giving things in Cobargo, one guy came, and his car was filled with bottled water from Aldi. He told Chris, 'I'm sorry I couldn't bring this till now, but I didn't get paid till yesterday.' Now there's somebody who lives from week to week, so if a very wealthy person sees this, sell some of your houses.

Build some houses for homeless women over 55 or for those suffering from domestic violence. Put some programs in place to stop men from committing violence. Help them understand why they don't need to. Put something into the grassroots community and help the grassroots people who have nothing but give everything.

Return to being kind and do unto others as you would have others do unto you. Buy somebody some flowers today.

The other thing I've done for 30 years, and you can do too. Now I'm old; I get away with it. People don't think I'm weird if I pass anybody anywhere, and they look pretty, their hair or nails are nice, or they've got lovely shoes on, and I say to them, 'Gosh, you look gorgeous today.' People love it.

Many years ago, we were going to the cinema over in Neutral Bay, and we passed this old couple, likely not as old as me now. She looked beautiful, and he looked so proud. I said to her, 'You look so beautiful.' Her face lit up, and after the cinema came out, we were walking back to the car, and he looked at me with such love in his eyes, and he said to me, 'Thank you,' and her face lit up.

It doesn't take much, does it? And the other most important thing is not to wear black. Black is for the devil. Put some colour on. Every day I go out, even if it's only to the supermarket, I'm beautifully dressed. I might have had the dress for 20 years—that's the one good thing about being a hoarder.

I've got yellow nails, and you have no idea how many times people say, 'I love your nails, I love your jewellery, I love your dress.' It lifts people's spirits. And do not wear black.

I have these wonderful helpers come, and I've had this gorgeous 24-year-old Belgian girl, very sweet and innocent. She said to me the other day, 'Margaret-Anne, have you always been this dynamic?'

I looked at her and said, 'This is somebody who's got to have a sleep in the afternoon. Do you still think I'm dynamic?'

She said, 'Yes, you are so dynamic. Have you always been like this?'

I said, 'I've got no idea. I'm always like I am now.'

But I thought out of the mouths of babes, we ought to see ourselves as others see us.

Lastly don't forget—do not wear black!

MARGARET-ANNE HAYES OAM

TERRY JAMES

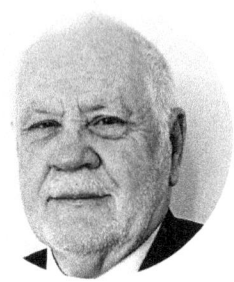

Terry is an early baby boomer. His life plan to become an archaeologist changed when he was conscripted into the Australian Army in 1966. He shares some of his traumatic experiences as an elite soldier. After two years, he left the army, became an accountant, and put the military out of his mind.

Over time, the memories flooded back, and he had to give up his job.

He eventually received help through the Department of Veterans Affairs and saw a psychiatrist for five or six years. He realises that you cannot go through a war and not be affected for the rest of your life. He will never lose his connections with his army friends.

He became involved with the RSL for some time and with several other community activities. He has a happy life with his three families, his own family, the army, and friends from school.

He has two children and five grandchildren.

My story starts on the fifth of June 1947, which makes me one of the early baby boomers. My mother was 29, and my father was 40. They met in World War II and had my sister Anne 12 years later. Sadly, I don't see her very often these days.

I was raised a Catholic and went to St. Patrick's boarding school in Goulburn passing the Leaving Certificate there in 1964. I've always wanted to be an archaeologist because I won the school prize for ancient history. I thought, I'll work for a couple of years, save some money, travel to England, go to Liverpool, go and see the Beatles at the Cavern Club and Carnaby Street in London, all those fabulous places of the early 60s.

I worked for a couple of years. Then, in 1966, I got this letter from the federal government: 'We want you for two years of military service.' I was conscripted into the Australian Army and entered on the fourth of October 1967. I was a soldier for two years. Knowing the things I know now I could have got out of it if I wanted to. But I didn't as it was the thing to do in those days. I felt some kind of duty, and even though with hindsight you look and think it wasn't the right thing to do. Should we have been there in the first place?

But that's how it was in those days, and I could cope with that.

I went through my three months of recruit training at Kapooka at Wagga, the only training centre. That was tough, but I was fortunate, as I'd been to boarding school for three years, it helped me interact with situations where I needed to look after myself.

When you graduate from the recruit training centre in the army, you have three choices of corps. I was a bit lazy and wanted to go to the armoured corps artillery or engineers. I applied for those and got the infantry. At the time, they just wanted bodies for Vietnam.

I was sent to Singleton for corps training and then posted to the Fifth Battalion Royal Australian Regiment based at Holsworthy. At that time, there were nine battalions in the Royal Australian Regiment, and I was in the fifth. Our mascot was a tiger.

I served in Australia for six months, then went to Vietnam from late January 1969 until October that year. After two years, I was discharged. I thought about staying, but I decided not to.

I still wanted to be an archaeologist, but there was no money in archaeology then, so I thought, okay, I'll study something where there's good money.

I started accountancy, which is boring but good money. I thought I might get back to archaeology one day, but I never did.

I've done accountancy since I left the army and am now retired.

I still love to watch ancient history shows on Foxtel and the History Channel, especially Ancient Egypt; it's my thing. However, it drives my wife insane because she hates it and loves movies.

Some of my youth was misspent. My three years of boarding school were wonderful, and I made some great friends. Before boarding school, I made a friend at primary school when I was five. I've got a photo of him at my fifth birthday party.

After being posted to the army, I walked onto the parade ground at Holsworthy and bumped into that friend whom I hadn't seen for ten years. I've known him for 70 years, longer than anybody in my family, even my sister, who is 12 years younger than me. Knowing someone for 70 years is a big thing. It makes me feel good to see him.

The army was great until I went to Vietnam. You make the best friends in the world, after the family, in the military. As I said, I didn't want to be in the infantry. I wanted to ride around in a Centurion tank or another personnel carrier.

Now, I am so proud that I was one of the elite infantry soldiers of the Australian Army; I get to wear my lanyard, which is in the War Memorial display case of the Hornsby RSL Club. On the left-hand side, I get to wear what's called an Infantry Combat Badge. Nobody else gets to wear those but infantry soldiers. You can say that because you survived. There were a few occasions where I nearly didn't survive. We had some tough times in Vietnam. I was there for nine and a half months. The battalion was there for 12 months, but my two-year commitment was up.

I was at Delta Company, which was based away from our main battalion unit. We were on SAS Hill, Special Air Service Regiment Hill, so we had a bit of privacy, which was good. We'd go out on operations for four to six weeks at a time, then back in camp for four to five days, then go out again, depending on the operational time, which varied from anywhere from a week to six weeks.

If you look through the history of that war, you find that the soldiers spent more time on the frontline than any soldier in any war that Australia has been involved in. It might not have been as intense as the trenches in World War I, but it was certainly more time on the front line. That's what we are told anyway and what we pass on to our friends and associates. They know that true story.

I had nearly got killed on many occasions, so I was lucky to survive. Ever since I got back when I was 22, I have felt good about surviving and being lucky.

There were two occasions where I nearly didn't survive. One was the battle of Long Tan. That's the first place I killed someone. It's not a nice feeling, but you don't think about it when you're shooting somebody in the back as I did. You just do those things. We sprung an ambush. In war, you have to do what you have to do to survive. At the time, it didn't affect me. But it took a long time to get back to what happened.

In the same operation, I lost a good friend who was killed. We used to have forward scouts, two forward scouts in each section, and you'd alternate. One day, you'd be the scout. The next day, the other scout would be in the front. One day, it was my turn to be at the front. And my friend said to me, 'I'll take it again today.'

I said, 'It's my turn; I'll do it.'

We walked into an ambush, and he got hit badly. He died five metres in front of me. After four hours, I couldn't get to him. I've always had a bit of survivor guilt because of that fact. He was a good friend. Sadly, he was due to go home the following week for the birth of his first child.

Circumstances like that are tough, but you go on because you have to go on. It's kill or be killed in war. That's what it's all about.

Another incident was the battle of Binh Ba, which took place after Long Tan. Binh Ba was a village well known for its rubber plantations and processing. It was a French village originally and quite a big town by Vietnamese standards.

One day, our battalion got a call from the village chief saying they had been overrun by the North Vietnamese Army (NVA) and Viet Cong (VC) and asked if we could come out to help. Normally, in a company, you'd have about 120 men. We had about 70–75 men because people were away on rest and convalescence, wounded, or doing courses elsewhere.

We were bundled into armoured personnel carriers and quickly driven out there with support by helicopter gunships and Centurion tanks. We spent three days house to house fighting in the battle of Binh Ba. It was something we weren't trained for; we were trained for jungle warfare. Fortunately, we only lost one person. It was very stressful; I can't remember much about it. I remember everything about my tour in Vietnam except those three days.

It was so intense. It really had an impact on me that I hadn't realised for a long, long time. I try to think back now, but I can't remember anything about what I did. Apart from the end of it, when we had to drag bodies into the central square, hundreds of bodies of what we called the enemy, VC, NVA, and regular army.

I had no recollection; I remember going there and leaving. We were in combat, going door to door. We had to evacuate most of them, but they also had cellars. It was house-to-house fighting, and the Viet Cong didn't have uniforms, so you couldn't tell who the enemy was most of the time.

The local Vietnamese cleaned a swimming pool that we used. One night, in an ambush, we killed some VCs, and one of those VCs was the swimming pool attendant. You couldn't tell who was friend or foe, just like the young guys in Afghanistan faced over recent years. You can't win the war against terrorists and insurgents by fighting cleanly. I wouldn't like to tell you what we had to do. I won't tell anybody that. My family knows nothing. We just talked amongst ourselves.

It happened the day after my 22nd birthday. I thought it was going to be my last birthday. It turned out not to be. I was very fortunate. It was very close on many occasions, but we survived. That was what got me going over there, house to house, fighting up close and personal with bayonets. You don't see much about that in the press these days. They fought bravely, as did we.

It changed my life a lot, but not immediately. I got home from war and tended to put it out of reach of everything or just completely forgotten about everything.

We were young—I came home at 65 kilos—and fit and healthy. Our brains might have been a bit addled when we got back for a while. Eventually, they wore away, but not completely—they never do.

I was discharged. We came home, went to North Head, and had to come in every day for a week. They put us on parade and called our names out; then we could go away and come back in the afternoon. That was it. At the end of that period, we signed a document. Instead of calling me Private James, which I was at the time, when you are called Mr James by an officer, you realise you're out of the army.

What do I do now? Before joining the army, I worked as a bus conductor for a year, trying to save money to go to England. But conscription ruined that, so I went to work in the bus depot for a while as I looked at what I wanted to do. I was collecting all the money, which I guess led partly to my interest in accounting.

Then I applied to join the Commonwealth Public Service and joined the Overseas Telecommunications Commission, where I worked for 11 years while I studied accounting. Over the years, I graduated from the Institute of Technology and worked in major corporate entities like Lifesavers confectionery, Cadbury, and several building companies. I worked as an accountant for a long time.

I still put Vietnam behind me to a certain degree. I made my life, put everything military-wise to the back of my mind, and forgot all about it. I kept working for a few years. Then, I fell apart at work.

I got married when I was 31, and that lasted seven years, but unfortunately, she couldn't cope with the stress I was going through. She was worried about Agent Orange[1] particularly with children and all that kind of stuff, so we eventually got divorced.

I'd given up on all the friends I'd made in the army and hadn't seen anybody, even my best friend, Gary Smith, a lovely guy. He got in touch with me and said, 'You're not doing very well. Why don't you go to the VVFA veteran's support centre at Granville and try and get a war service pension?'

I saw them and applied through the Department of Veterans Affairs. They were very helpful, and I was lucky because I was falling apart and had to give up my job. I didn't know what to do. All the memories came flooding back: good memories, bad memories, you name it, so I had to retire. I applied for a TPI pension from the Veterans Affairs Department, and I got that as I was a bit of a wreck.

I wasn't expecting that. When I came back from Vietnam, my mother said I had turned into a hard, cold person, which I think you've got to do. When you're 22, you're new to this. Is that real or not? War changes you.

I had a major nightmare probably about 15 years ago that a bayonet was thrust into my chest very slowly. I jumped up, screaming in the middle

---

1   Agent Orange was a powerful herbicide used by the US Army during the Vietnam War to eliminate forest cover and crops in the North. It contained dioxin, later proven to cause cancer, birth defects and severe psychological and neurological problems.

of the night. I remember that vividly. And I gradually weaned myself out of those. I don't know how, but I did, so I don't have those much anymore.

I dream here and there about military service. You can't be involved in a war that's kill or be killed and not think about it for the rest of your life.

I met the love of my life, Lyn, in 1987, and we're still together. She was recently divorced with two kids, Susan, 17, and Stephen, 14. Sue's now 53, and Steve just turned 50. That was tough at first; I didn't want to try to replace their father, and I just had to be a friend. That's what I tried to be. It was easy with Sue because she was all set in her ways; she was a teenager and left school, and Steve was still at school at that stage.

Now, I'm Pop to their children. Sue has three children. I love being Pop. I couldn't think of anything better in life than being a grandfather, even though it's not by blood; it's by heart.

It's been great that Lyn is five years older than me, and she's lovely; we are just made for each other. Meeting Lyn gave me a new lease on life and the love in my life; her family is mine, which I love.

We didn't want to have any kids straightaway, and because of the potential Agent Orange issues, she had one abortion because she didn't want to have the child because of that problem. We were engaged then, but we weren't married. I wanted the child, and I regret it now. But that happened. You can't change history, so I did not have any kids of my own.

Then I started seeing a psychiatrist which continued every month for about ten years. I gave that up a couple of years ago. I contacted my army friends and remade those contacts again. I'm involved in the RSL and ex-service organisations. I never wanted to be an RSL member when I got out of the army, but in about 1996, my best friend Gary talked me into getting involved in the RSL, which I did. I got heavily involved, then elected as Honorary Secretary of the Hornsby RSL sub-branch for five years, and then I was elected President of the Hornsby RSL for five years, which I gave up three years ago. I was heavily involved in the RSL in New South Wales. I was also responsible for organising all the Anzac ceremonies. I was on the National Committee for the Centenary of Anzac.

I was involved with the RSL for many years, and to a certain degree, I still am. Hopefully, I will become an attendant at the Cenotaph in Martin Place in Sydney in the next couple of weeks.

Where I am now is mostly in a happy place. I've given up seeing psychiatrists; I don't need to do that anymore. I'm not on any anti-depressant tablets.

My friend Gary, who has passed away, got me involved in golf 23 years ago. I've been playing every week for 23 years at Fox Hills, which is at Seven Hills Way, a long way from Asquith, where I live. But it's worth the trip because I love it. It's a great place to be.

I think I have softened a lot over the years. My involvement with Lyn and the kids and the grandkids they have helped make me a better person than I was. I was never really in trouble. I just was a cold, hard person. The sad thing about it was Mum died 12 years ago at 96 from dementia. She did not know me in the end. I'd like to think that she would have known me as a better person because of what I've done.

My next best group of friends are from boarding school because I spent three years at Goulburn, freezing in winter and hot in summer. But you made great friends here, too. We see each other regularly with what's called the Sydney Chapter. It makes me so happy that the young guys think enough of us to participate with us in what we do and enjoy our company. Everybody I know who is still alive comes to Sydney in December for a Christmas function, which is great.

I was giving a speech a couple of years ago at Hornsby Heights Public School. I spoke to the whole school. Then they asked me to go and speak in Year Four, they're about eight or nine, and one of the boys said, 'Mr James, what kind of gun did you have?'

I said, 'Oh, you probably wouldn't know, but it was a black one.'

'Oh, it was it an M16?'

They know.

Then, walking out the gate, a young kid who was probably about five or six years old, just in primary school looked at me and said, 'Mr James, I think you must have served in the army like my great-great-grandfather.' Potentially your great-grandfather. Perceptions of age. I love speaking to schools and do that regularly, though not as much as I used to. I'll leave that to somebody else; I did my bit. I still like speaking at schools and social community organisations.

I live in a townhouse at Asquith. I was a chairman of the strata plan for a while. I also gave that up, but I'm still on the committee. It's a great place to live. The people next door are a lovely family; they bring meals to us occasionally. We have drinks in the driveway on Saturdays and Christmas and Halloween functions there. It's a great community place.

My recollections and reflections on life are pretty good, I think. I don't ignore emotional issues anymore as I did for a long time. I didn't know I even had emotional issues.

The army became my second family; I will never lose the connection with my army friends. Over the years, I've given speeches at many schools and community organisations. Even though I'm not involved as president of the RSL anymore, I help keep the significance alive during the Anzac and Remembrance Day periods and all those kinds of events.

I've always tried to tell young kids these days that war is not good. It started with politicians but was fought by young men who committed their lives to war, so they should do everything they could to prevent future wars. Sadly, I don't think that wars will stop in this world. So, it's one of those things that I was trying to convince young kids to do. I told the kids there was negligence. Good people get killed, and horrible people survive. Who knows what will happen in the future, so you've got to try and prevent war as best you can in the world.

When I catch up with other war veterans, to be honest, I've never met anybody who doesn't have nightmares and flashbacks. They had issues. Agent Orange was a big issue at one stage. But I don't know many people who are affected by Agent Orange. Most people I know were affected by PTSD like I was. Because I had that survivor complex when my friend got killed instead of me, and we killed people. You think, I killed somebody. It's not right.

With wonderful hindsight, we should not have been in Vietnam. There was a time when there was a mentality in the world to stop the yellow hordes from coming south and support our allies, the Americans, who then asked to help the South Vietnamese; it carries on like that, right? Nobody should have been there; it's their country. Let them fight it out amongst themselves. But look at the war today; it's basically the same thing.

My life now is very happy. I've done a lot in the community but am cutting back now. I was treasurer of my golf club for a long time and on the board of the bowling club for a while. That's the kind of thing I've done a lot of the time. Everybody wants you to be a treasurer when they find you're a retired accountant.

When my youngest granddaughter, Charlotte, was around 10; she asked me to speak at her primary school for Anzac Day, which I did. She wrote a note about my situation and said, 'My pop served in the army, was in Vietnam blah, blah…' But the best thing she said was, 'I love him because he gives time to me all the time.'

That's the most important thing from my point of view. Even though they are not my natural grandchildren, my grandchildren love me. We're trying to say to the girls. 'Come on, girls, we want great-grandchildren, come on.'

My daughter says, 'We want to have grandchildren, Dad.' My son calls me Pop, and he's 56.

Like I said, we've got three families, family one at home. Family two, Army. Family, three boarding school, we see each other a lot. It's in the heart.

What I'd say to anyone who has been a soldier at war is *Duty Done. To the Regiment.* You can't say much more than that.

I never got wounded; I came quite close to dying many times. But I was fortunate. I have health issues now and then, but I don't complain because that's life. There are many people worse off than me in the world.

How lucky am I? Ever since I got home from war, I've been thankful from day one. I can't say more than that.

ALEX BRANDT

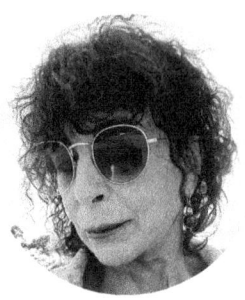

Alex's parents were displaced WWII refugees from Europe, eventually moving to Australia, where Alex was born in the 1960s. She faced cultural and language barriers growing up.

Alex missed the early formative years because she started school at eight and a half. She attended irregularly, faced integration challenges, and was labelled as a slow learner. This led to significant educational hardships.

Introduced to narcotics in high school, Alex used substances to cope, which led to deeper addiction issues. Despite this, she completed her secondary education and enrolled in TAFE.

Immersed in drug culture, Alex moved to a communal farm and later Sydney's Kings Cross, where she faced addiction, crime, and survival struggles. She experienced close bonds as well as significant losses.

Alex endured trauma from losing partners to drugs and being arrested for criminal activities. A pivotal arrest and subsequent miscarriage marked rock bottom for her and propelled her towards change.

Determined to reinvent herself, Alex pursued her education, acquiring forensic medicine and mental health degrees. She focused on understanding trauma and healing.

Alex now travels globally, sharing her story of survival and transformation. She runs a private practice, has written a book, and enjoys her role as a grandmother to her five grandchildren.

I'm grateful to share my story because it helps me reflect and see how the journey started and how it all unfolded.

My parents came here from Europe after the Second World War. My father was born in Odessa, Ukraine, while my mum grew up in the Baltic provinces in Europe. They both ended up in Germany as displaced refugees after the Second World War and came here to Australia. I was born here in the 1960s.

My parents were traumatised from their past and were carrying an awful lot of unresolved baggage. To put my story in context, it's easy for me to talk about it now because I've got the benefit of hindsight, but my parents were very shut down. They could not understand the culture and what was happening here or speak English.

English is not my first language, so I didn't speak English until I was about nine or ten years old, but they enrolled me in school when I was seven and eleven months old.

School, for me, was a very overwhelming place. Firstly, I didn't have the correct uniform because my mum didn't understand the concept of everyone wearing the same uniform, so I stood out from day one. Plus, I didn't speak English and had never been in a social setting before, so it was very difficult for me. Even my lunch was very different from everyone else's, so everything about going to school was uncomfortable.

But the worst thing that happened at that school was that there was a paedophile who worked as a janitor, and he is the reason, I guess, for the beginning of my intense trauma. After the abuse, I came home and told my parents, and then a big argument broke out between them, and they kept on arguing.

I was asked to go back to that school for three months before they took me out. By then, I had turned eight and was completely shut down. They took me to a doctor. In a sense, the doctor sides with my parents, advising them to never speak of this again and that the child, now eight, would forget about it. Finally, they did take me out, but after three months there, the damage was profound.

I was desperately unwell, shut down and confused. I had no structure because there was no school for me without any explanation. I think it's one thing being abused, but how it's received is a whole different story because that in itself is a trauma.

I have siblings, including a brother who is two years older than me and was performing very well, so I was compared to him. Roughly about the time they took me out of school at eight, my mother had my sister, so she's seven years and eleven months younger than I am.

My mother was busy with the new baby, and I became almost a problem in the family. My parents both decided that I was the problem, making their life even harder. That's how the scene gets set and plays out throughout the rest of the time. They took that position, and that's how it stayed.

I was enrolled in a new school at eight and a half, so now I had a big gap. When I had the gap, I started wandering around the street during the day. I met other children who were also displaced or wandering. Somehow, they weren't at school either. That started my journey, where I felt I was no longer part of the family and was drifting.

When I returned to school, I had to learn English. The school environment was very triggering for me, and I could not settle, learn, or get on with the children at school.

A different story developed from there, and I went to primary school until year four. I was put into years one, two and three, which I didn't complete, but they keep putting me up. Then, in year four, I'm taken out and don't appear back on any school roll until high school.

I was 12 or 13 when I started high school. By then, I'd been speaking English, but I'd basically been learning nothing. I couldn't read or write, and I was labelled as a slow learner, difficult and perhaps someone who couldn't learn. I remember the headmistress talking with my mum and saying, 'Alexandra might be better off not attending school at all and working in a factory because that's all she may be capable of.'

But I managed to stay in high school. In my later years of high school, there was a male teacher who befriended me and started driving me home and befriending me and talking to me about his marital problems. By then, I had accepted my role as a different person, a young teen who didn't belong. When I told my mother about this, she said, 'You are the problem, and all these things are happening to you because it is your fault.'

I did pass the HSC, although not very well. But in high school, the young teens among I was mixing with were two sisters who were using a narcotic drug. That was my introduction to this substance, and when I used it, everything in my life—every problem—disappeared completely. I felt emotionally relieved, and it felt like magic. I had no pain. It's funny that when I look back on that, I didn't feel that I was in pain, but I only noticed it when I started using the substance and was emotionally pain-free.

It helped me complete school. I spoke to my parents in a respectful tone and was able to live at home because of the substance that was helping me. Even though I did not do very well in my HSC, I was determined to keep going. I enrolled in a TAFE course equivalent to the HSC at Ultimo TAFE, where I had a completely different experience. There were adults doing that course, and the teachers were completely different. In that whole year, I caught up with my six years of high school.

I got a scholarship to either go to New South Wales Uni or Riverina College of Riverina for a teacher scholarship and chose Riverina because it was my way of getting out, of escaping.

'Doing a geographical' in mental health terms, that's what it's called.

When I got to Riverina College, I found that I was eligible to do other courses and other subjects. Maybe because I needed to work out what was wrong with me, I chose psychology. I was enrolled in a psychology course while using a narcotic. I attended very briefly. I started the course, then realised it was way over my head, and I could not do it.

I left college and moved out to a place called Riversdale, on the edge of Wagga. It's a hippie farm with other lost souls. Some are using, some are not, some are there because they like the lifestyle. I gravitated to the narcotic users, and we start living a lifestyle completely outside of society now. I've let the studies go. My family is completely estranged from me, and I'm in a world of using now. It keeps on going, this is where my life is headed now.

I felt connected to those people; we had a common goal. They were also broken and had their own stories, which I strongly identified with. It was almost calming and soothing for me to make those identifications and connections. We had our own solution, our secret. We had our own medication, and so, weirdly, it made sense for a short time. That's how the spiral began.

In the beginning, it seemed pretty innocent and quite freeing. We were not part of society; people were getting along and wearing very nice hippie clothes. There was music and a sense of community. However, the next thing that happened was the drug took over, and I saw my peers and my young friends overdosing and dying. That was an enormous reality shock for me, and for a short time, it startled me and pulled me up. But the promise of relief was so great. I was now seeking relief from the trauma of what was happening to me in the drug world.

I ended up on the streets of Kings Cross, the drug world of Sydney. The streets, the crime, the older addicts, and the experienced drug dealers. I was swamped, with nowhere to go except to somehow work it out. I had no idea how, but I knew I was not in the right place now and had fallen beneath society's norms to a huge degree and falling levels in myself. What didn't seem right the day before suddenly seemed the norm.

That sort of drug use also requires teamwork, where you team up with a specific person. The people I was teaming up with were men who were incredibly street-smart but had a criminal past. We become connected, and that's very treacherous because it involves violence, including domestic violence. There was continual pressure to keep producing ways of earning money to buy the substance because, by then, the substance had taken over. It had taken priority, and everything the group was doing was focused on the substance, but also knowing that we were all going to our deaths. It was obvious that people around us were overdosing and dying, and people around us were not coming out of this alive.

It was such a fast-moving, slippery slope, and the addiction was now jumping all over me. That's how it felt. I ended up being married four times, with three of those in the drug world. All those partners died while I was still in the group abusing. When one partner died, I ended up creating a new relationship with someone else. The lifestyle is so hard and harsh, and they die a desperate, horrendous death. That brought it home, even for me, that this is where I'm headed.

In a way, it was like everyone was in God's waiting room. Everyone is waiting, but at the same time, there is no way of coming back from that. That could be me. Anyway, yeah, so what.

What happened to me? I have met some other people this has happened to. It's where you fall way beneath your own level of coping. I was arrested with my last husband; he ended up suiciding after that. But we were arrested in Melbourne for a crime we did not commit.

When we ended up in the police station, the confession was already there in front of me; all I had to do was sign it. But I refused to sign it. The interview went terribly wrong. I was pregnant and handcuffed to the back of the chair, so I could not move.

The detectives turned on me. That wasn't unusual back then because we were seen as garbage. That's not an uncommon thing that happened on the street. The unusual thing was that they persisted with ferocity. The tragedy for me was that I had a miscarriage. I was so shocked that this could even be happening.

They could see what was happening to me, and they untied me and threw me into a cell. Now, when I put myself back in that place of the emotional pain, the powerlessness, the physical pain, the desperation, some people might call it rock bottom. People have described things like this as a moment of clarity. With that comes a knowing that it is done. I am over this. I am done. I described it like my toenails and hair knew it, and every part of me knew that was as far as I go.

The gift of desperation. With it comes a different type of strength, a different type of clarity, and an absolute knowing that it's over. I have seen the darkest moment, the most desperate time I needed to see or experience. I don't mean I needed it, but it was almost like the darkness now fell away.

That's what happened.

Making the darkness conscious. I felt, I sensed, I saw, I knew where I was and the horror of my own story and the horror of my position in the scheme of light. With that came an incredible wisdom and knowing, and it happened fairly quickly, but I knew to the bottom of my being that that was it for me. I wasn't going to destroy my life. I wasn't going to destroy another human's life. I'm going to make it count. I am now done with all of this. And that's how it happened.

One of the platforms that I have used is education. I went back through school. I went through university. I did forensic medicine at university. I did a degree called accredited mental health social work. I also did 15 years of language studies, where I went back to culture and looked at language studies. I've done many years of studying war and the trauma of war.

What does war do to people's self, like their psychology? What's the psychological impact on a person who's gone through the Second World War or Vietnam or Korea? Every war has its own psychological stamp of trauma.

I went back to look at what had happened to my parents. I felt close to their roots and wanted to retrace my family lineage. I've needed to find a deep level of forgiveness and gratitude for a big part of this reconstruction and transformation. Knowledge is power, and knowledge has been something I've used in my process of reconstructing myself.

These days, I'm so passionate about not hiding the flaws, but I am so passionate about seeing the cracks. About showing who we are, not for instance, as a woman, but as a man as well, as a soul that's been completely and totally broken and then can rebuild and reconstruct itself in a new way and then look back. Like a butterfly that emerged from a caterpillar, as someone once said, it never looks back in shame on the chrysalis it popped out of. I love that.

I've got two beautiful daughters. They've had five children between them, so I'm a grandmother. I've written a book. Now, I have a private practice and do a lot of travelling. I have been involved in giving talks.

I've been to Russia several times and the Ukraine before the war, of course, and I saw where my father grew up. I'm travelling to Cyprus in a month, where I'll be involved in some talks and meetings about people who are also seeking transformation and have been to the depths of their own rock bottom.

What I learned along the way are transferable skills, so we can use them to survive. But on the other hand, we need to use them in a very different way. One thing that was very difficult for me was I had to let go of the person who survived the trauma, the person who survived my own personal war, and let the real person emerge.

It's very difficult to let that go because that was the person I depended on, the person who life made me. She had to let go of some of those beliefs and survival skills and then transform that and become who I was, should have been, could have been; my authentic self underneath all that.

If this is you, I suggest you get in touch with your authentic self. Who am I really? The authentic self seems to be the child. It was an enlightening moment for me when I realised that is who I am.

It's then about finding different methods of reparenting yourself and bringing her out of the shadows, not abandoning her, being there for her, and following all that up.

Then it's an internal love story, if you like, of acceptance.

ALEX BRANDT

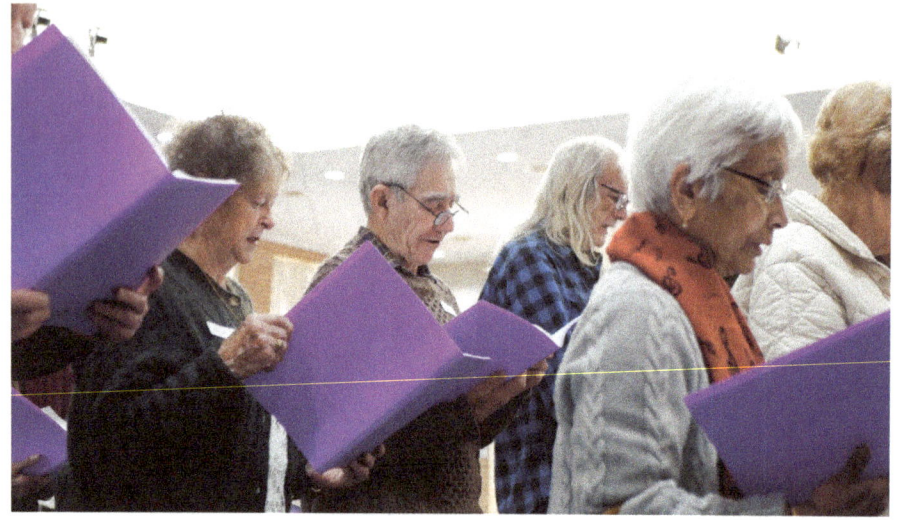
Community Choir CourtesyBernardo Winck

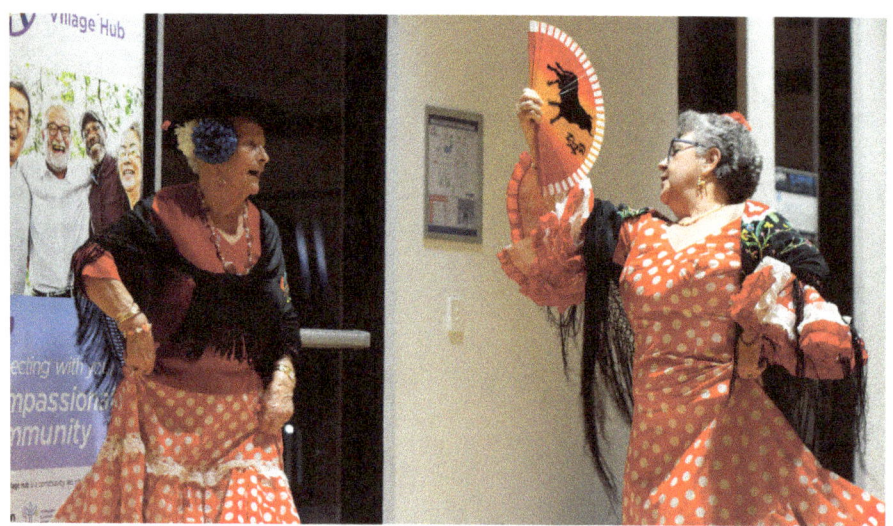
Multicultural Event Courtesy Marilia Gauche

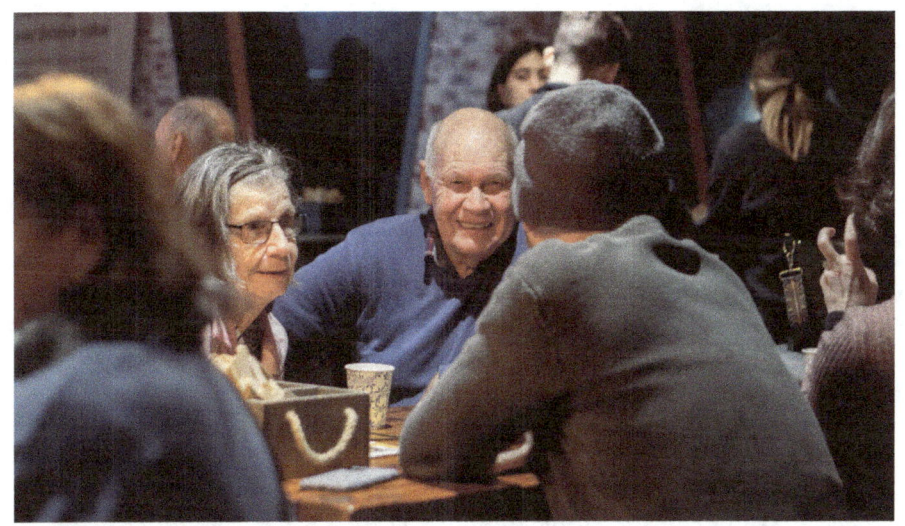

Our Stories Matter Courtesy Marilia Gauche

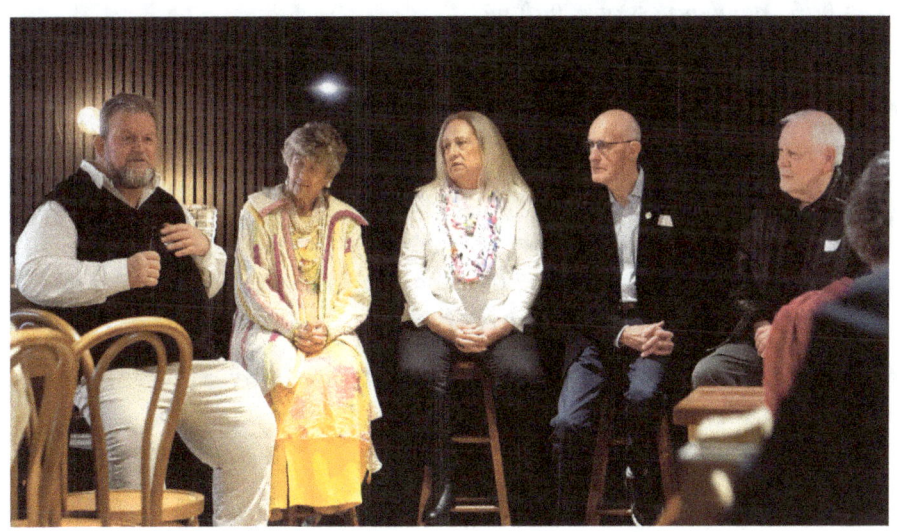

Our Stories Matter Courtesy Marilia Gauche

BRADLEY DOWLING

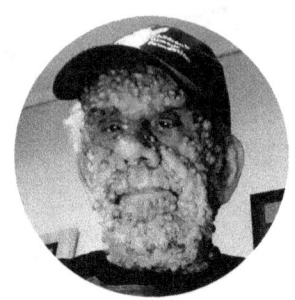

Bradley Dowling, now 65, was diagnosed with neurofibromatosis at age 5, so he faced a lifetime of physical and social challenges. His condition affects his skin, causing visible tumours. Despite heartaches and staring from others, his positive outlook and authenticity made profound impacts, emphasising openness over judgment.

Bradley has spent 28 years as a support worker, primarily aiding individuals with cerebral palsy in New South Wales. His empathetic approach provides essential support, helping people pursue activities and achieve their goals despite disabilities.

Bradley teaches scripture in schools and is involved with chaplaincy, merging his passion for faith with education. Alongside attending church, this role enriches his life with purpose and spiritual fulfilment.

Bradley found joy in coaching 'leftovers,' kids overlooked by other teams. His efforts brought them confidence, leading to victories and even new responsibilities like refereeing.

Deeply invested in the neurofibromatosis community, Bradley works to raise awareness and support for those affected. He is a member of the Children's Tumour Foundation of Australia. He shares his experiences to reduce stigma, helping others navigate their conditions with better understanding and community backing.

BRADLEY DOWLING

Emphasising fitness and healthy living, Bradley leads by example. His involvement in activities like the Ocean Beach Surf Club underlines the importance of physical health and an active lifestyle, furthering his overall well-being and capacity to help others.

I'm from Mt Colah. I've got two brothers and a sister. One brother lives on Norfolk Island, and another brother lives off the coast of Cairns on Fishery Island. My sister is down in Frenchs Forest. I have lived in other areas, but all roads always seem to come back to Mount Colah. This is a good area; we grew up here. I went to school at Mount Colah and Asquith.

We're in the quiet area of Mount Colah. We've got a bush view, and we look out, and there's nothing there; it's just all bushland and quiet and peaceful.

I have a condition called neurofibromatosis (NF), which is a genetic condition that affects various parts of the skin. I found out when I was five that I had the condition, and as years went by, the lumps grew onto the facial areas and the body area. Currently, I work with the Cerebral Palsy organisation. I've been doing that for 28 years as a support worker for disabled people, mostly Cerebral Palsy, in St Ives in New South Wales. I also enjoy coaching kids' basketball and attending church.

My goal and focus are to help promote neurofibromatosis and help people overcome their condition. Not one person has the same form of NF, which we'll describe as we go along.

I only work three days a week, Monday, Tuesday, and Thursday. I also teach scripture in schools, which I love. I do light exercises, keep fit, and maintain a healthy lifestyle.

I took up coaching and running basketball back in the nineties. In those days, the police youth club was in George Street in Hornsby, so I'd go in on Saturday morning to set up for the kids. We only had one court in those days, so we ran the basketball from early morning to early evening. We got to know many people as they came in with their families. My intention when I first took over wasn't coaching. They just wanted someone who could supervise children and run the competition.

There was a team with nobody to coach them, so I thought, I'll coach them. It's proving what other kids can achieve when no one else wants to ask them to give them a chance. It just fell into place, so the very first time I ever coached, we made the grand final.

If you can give them something they can believe in or do things, everything else falls into place. I never played basketball and had no idea. I was asked, 'Can you just coach them?' I enjoyed it. As men, we became very competitive.

I only coached the young men, always with the parents around, ensuring everyone knew what was happening.

The parents just needed someone to show them what to do. Over the years, I coached those who never had a coach or where they just had leftovers and kids who couldn't find a place in the team. Unfortunately, some kids were not wanted in a team, so I said, 'Give me the kids. I'll show you what we can do.'

I learned that you could give them confidence so they know someone believes in them and is there for them. Many kids would come in and be given an opportunity to achieve, and they enjoyed it. As time went on, as I was still supervising, we allowed kids to referee the games and do other things. They gained a lot of confidence. On Saturday mornings, I felt like I was a drop-in centre for people.

Well, it's a lot different now, but it's still a concept of helping them to believe, helping them to have confidence. It's how you communicate with them and how you can have conversations around sports.

Now I'm not doing basketball; I'm only going into the schools to do the scripture. But I'm grateful for that period I had at Hornsby, and then

I went over and did a few things in the Hills area. But Hornsby was where the door opened, and today, nearly 30 years later, I see some of the kids walking around with their kids.

I still get a grateful thanks for what we did. The kids always had to be focused, and right from day one, they needed to know where they stood. In other words, in classes, it's very simple. I talk, you listen. Anyone else in class talks, and everybody else listens. It's a simple way of saying this is what we need. This is what we focus on.

It's the same thing in basketball. You come in and you listen to what I say. I listen to what you say and was able to say three times, and you're out.

One of the things I am grateful for is that they took me for who I am. They saw me as being me, even with the skin condition; the kids never focused on that. One of the lovely comments I always get is, 'At first, when we talk and see you, we find it quite daunting, but afterwards, we don't notice your skin condition. We notice you.'

I'm always happy to tell them. I always say, 'If you want to ask, I can tell you, but I hate the stares and whispers.' People will stare, and they'll whisper.

There are a lot of challenges with the skin condition, and it's hard if I go to places where people don't know me, but it's okay if I'm around people who know who I am. There have been always challenges. People think you're always bright, happy and cheerful. But I do have my days with this condition, which can be pretty daunting sometimes.

You wish it would go away. Many people with NF won't go out in the community or won't be seen because of the fear of what people will say and what they'll do. Again, the cliché of stares and whispers.

I was at a men's breakfast a couple of weeks ago and turned around; this eight-year-old was looking at me and saying, 'Hello.' Dad was next to him, and I looked up and thought, oh, my goodness, it was a kid I coached nearly 30 years ago with his son.

He said, 'Can you do me a favour? This is my son and he's curious about it.' I said, 'Okay.' Because he knew about it and wanted his son to know about it too.

I said, 'I'll tell you what it's all about. This is the skin condition. I'll give you a little card, and you and Dad go home, and you can have a chat about it.'

It was just for him for his son to understand so that he knew about it; his dad could go home and explain that I helped him with basketball and stuff.

We picked up the importance of letting people know you can overcome what you can. And I've got the Christian faith to believe God gets me through. It's important to let kids know they or anyone I talk to can achieve.

Just one of the things is that never quit and never give up.

Last time someone asked me, 'Could I take your photo?'

And I said, 'Yeah, that's $50.'

One of the beautiful things for me is not to be afraid to do things. They wanted me to do it on the TV show. I said, 'I'm more than happy to do that.' I've been in magazines like Take Five, That's Life and a few other magazines and newspapers, sharing my story about my condition, overcoming adversity and being able to let people know. God's great gift is to do stuff and not be afraid to stand in front of people and talk.

It's the honesty about being who you are. Yes, there are difficulties, and yes, you've got to overcome them. If you can overcome, then you can keep going. People come and point. 'Look at that man.'

Many years ago, a little kid said, 'Hey, mister, how'd you get all those lumps?' I'm thinking, I didn't eat my green vegetables when I was your age.

It's an emotional challenge, but I've got good family support. My late dad, mum, brothers, sisters, and family always supported me and other good people around me who took me as who I am, like when I did children's ministry when I did kids' basketball or youth basketball. It's about being able to be who I am.

Well, as I said, when they discovered my NF at five, it was through café au lait spots, which look like coffee-stained spots. But as I got older, the lumps came on me. Doctors can operate. That's when it got more difficult. They take some of the lumps off, but they will always grow back.

But I'm thankful that the good Lord has helped me. I've done a lot of prayer and discovered that although God was always looking after me, my parents always were there. I found a reality God showed me: that I could do things for myself. An important thing is learning to trust in God and learning that I've got a verse I use; it's in the Psalms that says, 'I'm fearfully and wonderfully made, and my soul knows well.'

Being able to help people is one of the important things to me, as well as seeing things from another perspective and wanting to make someone achieve something. As I mentioned, I always had the team with the leftovers and kids with nobody to look after them or want to do it. It was important to let the kids share your journey and enable them to know that they can do things.

Many years ago, I had a team out at Castle Hill, and I asked the parents to give me two seasons. In the first season, we didn't win a game. I said, 'Let the kids stay here; believe me, we can do this.' Then, the following year, we won the grand final, so we went from last to first.

For the parents that have faith in me to trust the kids, when any parent trusts you, it's quite an honour and a privilege to say, 'All right, look after them, take care of them.'

One year, I had a basketball team, and I called on the leftovers. The kids didn't know each other when they came together. I said, 'You were in there, he was there, and you all came together.'

One of the kids said, 'I guess we were leftovers, weren't we?'

Working in the same job for 28 years with people with disabilities has been good. I've learned that we're the lucky ones; some people need help more than we need help, and obviously, the same goes with families or carers. Their trust is in you to look after them. This is more difficult because they have more special needs, so there needs to be much more time spent there. But you don't stay in the job if you don't enjoy it.

They've got to try, and again, like the able-bodied, you've got to give them the opportunity to do and achieve what they want. We have different activities. I run a group called Boccia, which is like an Olympic sport, but we do it in a fun way. Boccia is simple: blue ball, red ball, and jack. They've got to get as close as possible to the white jack. We have a bit of fun with that.

I'm in other groups at work, where we do activities, music, art, and other areas, but it's also about ensuring we can set goals for them. Some can't communicate vocally, so they might have other ways of communication. One of the things I've learned is not to feel ashamed of what you have and not to blame. It's never ever a blame game. Once you start having a blame game, then that's it. It's very important to know that one, don't blame. Two, just keep doing what you need to do.

I'm the only one that has NF in the family. No one else has it, and we don't know where it came from. NF can be what they call generations genetic. It's skipped a generation somewhere. I'm the one that's got it. Some people are much worse than me and unfortunately, the others with the NF can have a limb amputated because the condition can grow inwards and cause a lot of damage. You can have NF1, NF2. I'm NF1. I have more appearance. NF2 is inward. Mine's just more noticeable.

They said they wanted to do some genetic testing on my late dad and mum to find out, but I never told him. I could never put them through going to the hospital, and then suddenly, one of them discovered that they were carrying the NF gene. That's something that I always hold with me, and I never want anyone on that side to find out.

Dad passed away about six years ago. Mum is coming up to 95, and she's in aged care. But you cherish your parents and your family, and I am always thankful that I've got my family around me to help and support me and carry me through.

The interesting thing is going back to basketball after all these years, and how this has got me thinking is that in the last couple of weeks, a few times, I've got a tap on the shoulder from some of the old kids I've coached who are now adults. Some parents are saying, do you remember you used to coach my son all those years ago? I thought, Lord, you wanted me to go back to basketball?

I enjoy doing the scripture at school, so I do that on Wednesday mornings. I've got a class at Mount Colah and an assistant class at Mount Kuring-gai. But I think, generally, I'm also getting back on track with the NF association. Now, it's called the Children's Tumour Foundation of Australia. Many years ago, it was called NF Australia. I gratefully got the Ambassador of the Year award. I was the president of the association back in the heydays. Still, I was very grateful that Mum and Dad were involved, and they both received lifetime achievement awards.

But, come on, give me more interviews, more TV so I can share my story and my journey.

Going back to the kids coaching and taking the leftovers, I was always the last one picked on a team or never picked on a team. I was always the leftover, so I know what it's like for kids who are leftovers and to understand that they're on a journey, too.

There's a gentleman in his forties, and we catch up once every three to four months. He's married, with his wife and kids, and he was the first kid

I ever coached. Our families are connected, so we'll touch base every three to four months and say, 'How are you going? What's happening?'

He's the only kid, the first and only kid I ever told, 'I don't want you ever to play basketball.'

He was a very good soccer player and came to me one day and said, 'I've got a choice. Either I play soccer or play basketball.'

I said, 'What's your best chance of making reps? Basketball or soccer?'

He said, 'soccer.'

I said, 'Good, don't play basketball.'

He became a representative in soccer and made the rep teams. The kids want to hear those kinds of things, he probably knew, but he wanted to hear it honestly and openly.

So, what do I love to do now? Well, I'm a member of the Ocean Beach Surf Club, so I'll go backwards and forwards every now and then. I've got the Children's Tumour Foundation; it's about just doing things.

I'm in a place now, at 65, where it's—what are you going to do? I've done all I wanted to do at work. I've had my share of heartaches, my share of breaks, and my share of stares, whispers, taunts, and things like that, but I'm still here.

BRADLEY DOWLING

NARELLE GATTI

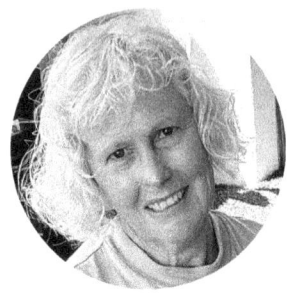

When Narelle was 42, her life changed forever when she lost her eyesight.

Since then, she and her family have had to learn to navigate life in a very different way.

Narelle grew up on a cattle property, and the resilience and skills she acquired there served her very well as she struggled to adapt and solve problems day by day.

'Because there are two things you can do in life. When you face an obstacle, you can turn it into a barrier and sit in the corner and cry. Or you can turn it into a challenge. Stand up and say, "Okay, how will I fix this? How am I going to do it?" I choose to make it a challenge and to laugh. Find the funny side in whatever it is. It is a choice, and I choose to get on with it.'

Narelle has been doing amazing things to help raise awareness for people who are struggling with disabilities.

'So, how do you treat people with a disability? Treat them like everyone else. To be honest, their disability is no one else's business.'

I'm a typical mum. When all this went down, my dad had died about 18 months previously. My three sons were in school between grades eight or nine, the youngest was in grade four or five.

My husband and I were both working. We lived in a suburb north of Brisbane where there wasn't much public transport; that's important for what happened. There was a train and buses about every half hour or so. We lived on a fair-sized block at the end of a cul-de-sac.

We were enjoying life. Most of my family lived out in the bush with no public transport. I would hop in the car at about 4:00 a.m. with the boys to visit my mum; we would drive about eight hours to Central Queensland. Mum was still driving at that stage. My sister was 11 hours away, also with no public transport. My older brother lives in Rockhampton, but he travelled out to our cattle property where I grew up. My younger brother also lived outside Rockhampton.

I worked in Brisbane in the public service. I'm a computer programmer by trade. Part of my work involved validation, which required looking at maps using a mapping tool called Esri. It was about validating networks, and I had to validate and test my code so that our results were correct. I could look at the maps and say, in essence, road A connects to road B. That's the basis of what we were doing at the time.

I had started that job only about three months previously when I began having car accidents, which really threw me. I thought, oh, that car suddenly popped up. You assume they were speeding.

Then I started falling over chairs, thinking, what's going on? I had a new pair of glasses, so I went to my optometrist, who also happens to be one of my good friends, and said, 'Lisa, I think we've got a problem with the glasses.'

She said, 'What do you mean?' I told her what happened, and she got me to do a visual field test. This tests if you can see where something is in space. It could be, for example, a tree over in the left corner.

But I had no fields. I could only see directly ahead, which is why I was having car accidents and falling over chairs and everything else. To all intents and purposes, I was legally blind. As I'd driven there, Lisa's husband went to get my husband. From that moment on, I was never allowed to drive again legally, which meant kids, sports, groceries, doctors, and everything else, all my activities as a wife and mum, had to change. Even getting kids to and from school.

I worked and did the cooking because I still had direct sight, but it explained many things. It also completely changed my husband's and kids' lives because they suddenly had to step up and be more responsible. My husband had to take over many of my jobs because I couldn't drive the kids to footy or cricket practice. I couldn't do any of it. There was no public transport, so it was impossible.

I have two autistic kids. It was, oh my gosh, what am I going to do? Getting dinner, getting the homework done, making sure the clothes are ready, all the usual mum stuff.

Afterwards I had to say to my husband, I can't remember which sport it was. 'The practice is on tomorrow. How are we going to get them there?'

If it was football, well, we only had one car. We used to drive to the one game with one kid, and we had two on one team and one on another. One parent would stay with that child, and the other would drive to wherever the other had to go. Now, we couldn't even do that.

We had to do a lot of problem-solving to try and fix the immediate problems very quickly to get through the next day. Then it was, 'What are we going to do the next day? Let's solve that one.'

We just had to break it down. Being analysts probably helped. But I didn't have the opportunity to grieve or anything because we had three kids. I was still Mum, he was still Dad, and we had to get them to what they needed to do.

We just had to problem-solve very quickly to get things done; it was hard. Looking back, I don't know how we did it. We just did it because we had no option.

Growing up on a property helped me. A friend once said, 'You're tough because your father was tough and tough on you.' We didn't have electricity when I was growing up. I was about 12 when we got electricity, so I was used to a wood stove, kerosene lamps, and generators. We used the kerosene lamp if we didn't have the generator on. We had kerosene fridges and heaters.

We didn't have a shop; the nearest shop only covered the basics. If you needed food, it was an hour away, so we made do. Mum grew the veggies. We had to ration water in the dry time. We had cattle. But you learned to make do because that's what we had.

Making do was probably our saving grace. We always had milk powder in the cupboard, so if we didn't have milk, we had milk powder.

Now, we had to do things like that. We would shop and always had the spare packet of wheat, or whatever it was. We started buying meat in bulk. We got a freezer because then we didn't have to worry about that so much. It was just easier. We bought bread and milk in bulk and everything we could. If Mark couldn't go shopping, it didn't matter because the food was there. We just had to change.

Doing that was going back to how I grew up. However, clothes are an issue because kids quickly grow out of their clothes. I couldn't get to the uniform shop at school, so I was reliant on friends. I would ring up my friend who was running the uniform shop. She'd ring me back and say she had paid it and what I owed her. That's how we had to do uniforms.

It wasn't just one thing, but it was everything. We had developmental paediatricians with our Aspergers boy. We had all the medical stuff that you have with kids. We had kids in braces, so we had to get around things. Back then, there was no NDIS and no support for what I was going through. You just made do and worked it out because you had no options.

We brought our kids up to be independent. We were determined that they would know how to clean, cook, and everything else, so by that stage, they knew how to cook and clean. We'd already said, 'If you're old enough to make a sandwich on a weekend, you're old enough to make your own lunch,' so they were making their own lunches.

The homework became an issue because Mark got home much later than me. I would catch the bus home, catch a train, catch a bus, and get home that way. Then I'd say to the boys that I could still see in front of me, but they had to take on just a lot more responsibility.

I was still doing the mowing and most things. However, the more sight I lost, the more they had to pick things up and just run with it. It's like night blindness; I really struggled at night. I would have the dinners cooked for the week. The boys would then have to cook veggies or rice or pasta, heat the meals up and set the table if they wanted to eat. They all stepped in. I'm so lucky. My husband stepped in with the shopping, the footy training, and the cricket; he just had to do it.

But it became too much. In the end, the kids didn't ever work outside the home because with only one person with a license having to go grocery shopping and do everything else, he couldn't then drive them to a job, pick them up, and all those things. They never had those opportunities, and it impacted them. But they learned a lot of other skills they never thought anything about.

In order to attend the parent-teacher meetings, I had to take the day off from work and catch the school bus with the kids. They hated it, and so did the other kids, because I knew a few of the parents and the bus driver. It wasn't the biggest suburb, so I knew the people and the teacher would meet me at the school, and off we'd go.

Kids are resilient. We'd already taught them how to think outside the square, make do, and be resilient, although they worked out how to talk their way out of things at school at times. But that was their choice and consequence; they had to live with that. They knew what they had to do.

It was really hard. I had to keep telling myself that. We'd always taught them, especially my Asperger's son, that there's more than one way to skin a cat or do something. Just because I can't do it one way doesn't mean there's not another way.

For example, when sweeping a floor, I would start missing bits because I didn't realise I was missing them, so we got a better vacuum cleaner. Then I would take a step—vacuum around that area—take a step. I had to relearn. It was the same with cooking.

I don't know how many times I've relearned how to do everything. But in the end, I had a saying, *'If I don't mind, it don't matter.'* Then, I had to convince myself that I didn't mind.

It came down to me saying, well, I've got to do it. I am still a mum and very much a wife. Those two roles are very important to me. I am a daughter, sister, and friend, and those roles are also very important to me, so if I wanted to be there and have those people in my life…

Don't get me wrong. I cried a lot in the shower, but not in front of the boys; it was in my private time. I used to say to the boys, 'Get over it. Get on with it. You've got to live.'

When the boys were at school, I'd ring my mum, my sister Jude, and my closest friend, Jude. They became my saviours. I would start to have panic attacks, and I'd ring my sister, and she would say, 'Right, let's start breathing.' Then we breathed through it, and I'd say, 'Right, I can do it now.'

If I couldn't get my sister, I'd ring my friend Jude, and she'd say, 'It's okay. Come on, stop it. Don't be stupid. Get on with it.' Then came the day when my friend Jude rocked up to my place and said, 'Sit down. I'm dying. I'm not going to be here in six months, so losing your sight is nothing. You will be taking on my girls as well now.'

I said, 'Yes, they're my girls.' They are still my girls. All the six kids accept disability. One of the girls has a lot of disability, and she's also been taught to get on with it.

The two Judes, my mum and my husband got me through. My husband would give me a hug and say, 'It'll be alright. Get over it. It'll be right.'

There are two things you can do in life. When you face an obstacle, you can turn it into a barrier and sit in the corner and cry. Or you can turn it into a challenge. Stand up and say, 'Okay, how will I fix this? How am I going to do it?' I choose to make it a challenge and to laugh. Find the funny side in whatever it is. It is a choice, and I choose to get on with it.

So, how do you treat people with a disability? Treat them like everyone else. To be honest, their disability is no one else's business.

Don't ask them things. I have a guide dog, and I'm often asked, 'Are you training the dog?'

I'll say, 'No, he is my guide dog.'

'Oh, are you blind?'

There are degrees of blindness, so I say, 'Yes.' It's simpler.

Go up and say 'G'day, how are you going?' Don't stare. Say your name so I know who I'm speaking to. If you just say, 'Hi, Narelle,' I might not want to talk.

My biggest thing is don't assume anything. A person could be just having a really bad day and may need time out, so they might just nod and keep walking. It's not rudeness; you don't know what's going on in their life. They might be deaf and can't hear you anyway. It could be that they have their mind on something else entirely and didn't notice you. Or they are incredibly shy or have anxiety.

There could be so many reasons, but we are all normal. Everyone is normal. The person who has no hair is normal. A person with a big nose is normal, and a very tall is still a normal person with feelings. If you're in a room with them, say, 'Hi, I'm so and so. How are you going today? How's your week been?' Normal conversation. If they choose to tell you, they'll tell you. If they don't choose to tell you, that's fine.

I've started a podcast called the Digital Access Show, and it's related to everything I do now. It tells people about the digital accessibility standards, which are maintained by Standards Australia. It also tells us how to set up all the digital content so that most people, regardless of ability, can access the information and read and understand it.

It helps in so many ways with independence, with that mental lift, when you can be yourself and be independent and not have to ask someone to read it. Or to ask someone what they are saying because you didn't hear. These rules and guidelines are there, and they're backed by the Human Rights Commission, and the Disability Discrimination Act 1992.

We decided to set up a podcast around all of that, and the theme is communication, usability, and accessibility in the digital world. We talked to people about how they do things. A couple of weeks ago, it was this fantastic bloke called Patrick Dillon. Patrick is a disability employment specialist who also happens to be a quadriplegic and works full-time.

It's about how he uses the tools. We talked to Mark Muskett, who's never had sight. He is a digital accessibility trainer and travels Australia doing it. Alan Parker, who's dyslexic and a micro-behavioural neuroscientist and forensic linguist, travels the world teaching mediation negotiation, working as a negotiation specialist, and teaching communication. He loves neurolinguistics. Neurolinguistic plasticity is a big word there; it's awesome stuff.

Then there's Paula Burgess, who runs a business. She's also got an ASD son and the way that they work with him, and Grace Cameron, who has a disability called Postural Orthostatic Tachycardia Syndrome. POTS. She runs a business lying on a bed 23 hours a day; she can't stand for too long.

Adam Morris has no sight and works full time. He describes the tools he uses and the challenges he faces. Meryl Evans, who is hearing impaired, lives in the US and does what I'm doing. We looked at the differences between the US and Australia.

It's all about communication, how people communicate, and the digital tools that assist everyone. It really lets people know that they're not alone if they're struggling with whatever it might be.

They're not alone; there are so many people out there who are embarrassed, which is sad because they have no need to be embarrassed. They are who they are, and it comes down to accepting yourself. That's the hardest issue. Or they feel that other people just don't get it. But again, it's learning. That's the other person's issue—not theirs. They go out and are part of our society and our community because there are so many people in the world who want them.

Our podcast can also benefit the older generation. However, I would say to those people you've got the right to ask for the information in the form that you want. It is your right. If they say email address, you say, 'Don't have it; you need to send it to me on paper.'

They have that right and they should exert that right. There is no law that says you must have an email address if you don't want an email address. If you don't want a smartphone or feel that you can't use it, don't have it. Things can still be done on paper because it is your preferred communication style. If the business wants your money, then that is your preference. There is no rule.

If you have a disability, never be ashamed of yourself. Never be ashamed of who you are because of what you can do or what you need to do. Treat it as a challenge. It's never a barrier. Sometimes, you may have to ask for help, and I've asked for help many times, and I will do it again because asking for help is nothing to be ashamed of. It's saying you need to learn something different.

For everyone who doesn't have a disability, we're all normal people at the bottom.

NARELLE GATTI

IAN WESTMORELAND OAM

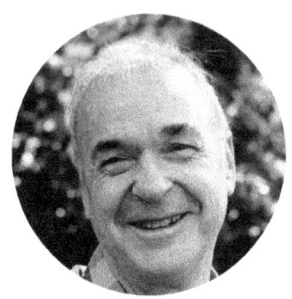

Ian, the founder of Kintsugi Heroes, tells his story as part of the Kintsugi Connecting to Seniors series.

However, this is about something other than Ian, who is well-practised at telling us how he became such an important person in creating organisations that support the community (you can find this information earlier in the book).

This is the story of Ian, a man of a certain age whose history brought him here to join our cohort of interesting older Australians.

It's funny; I struggle to think of myself as a senior, but I'm well and truly there, age-wise.

Overall, I view senior Australians as a huge, underutilised resource of wisdom and skills. Today, it's a lose-lose situation, an untapped potential. The negative mental and physical impact on those older people for being untapped creates many challenges around the lack of connection, support, and even respect.

There was an excellent TV documentary where they matched some of these older people with young kindergarten kids and then measured the various aspects of their physical and mental health. Like suicidal ideation or how long they could stand on one leg. It increased when they had this meaningful relationship with the young person.

I hear in the corporate world sometimes that there's too much grey, or a reluctance to recruit seniors, which I feel is not a sensible decision. I was fortunate to leave paid work when I turned 60 and start my own not-for-profit organisations. I wasn't dependent on someone looking at how much hair I had.

In Japan, there is far more respect for older citizens. In Europe, there is much more intergenerational interaction. My wife Helen's father was Italian, and in the Italian community, the seniors would often live with the family.

Australia has many negative traits, and hopefully, this project will help us address some of them.

Personally, I'd like to say I don't feel age has affected me, but that's not 100% truthful. I'm still incredibly active physically. I ride a bike around 140 km a week. On Tuesdays, I look after four-year-old and 18-month-old grandchildren. Then, I'm about five, mentally, running around, wrestling, and doing all this stuff.

But the reality is that last year, I thought I was going to die, and people around me thought I was going to die. I collapsed at home and finished up in hospital. I've been through a cancer recovery. So I guess that this is an indication of age but I'm feeling good now.

That was probably the wakeup call. I never see myself retiring. My wife says, 'You retired ten years ago.' I hate that and say, 'I didn't retire, I stopped paid work.' I want to continue to give back and to continue to learn until the day I die. That's where I'm at, and it is my mission.

Early in married life, the mission was to make money, as we were poor. Then, it became climbing the corporate ladder until the 10th of September 2013, when my life changed. Now it is a giving back mission of identifying and trying to live my best life. It certainly hasn't always been this way.

At times, it was totally appropriate to make money. You have to feed your family. We had our kids very close together, so, for many years, Helen couldn't work. My role was to put food on the table and get them clothed. Now, we're not wealthy, but I don't need to focus on that. I can do what I'm called to do in my mission for this stage; I don't want to say it, but it is the final stage of my life.

My wakeup call was actually three different illnesses. I had a cancer diagnosis and fortunately, there's a good prognosis now after a round of immunotherapy. There was another diagnosis of pulmonary fibrosis, which is a progressive, non-treatable lung disease. You lose the ability to breathe. I was upset that it would be this gradual decline, but it didn't feel right. I still don't believe it; I have a test coming up in a month.

The third one that knocked me for six was when I collapsed at home and finished up in Emergency at the hospital, feeling terrible. I managed to get out of the hospital as we had a book launch to do for Kintsugi Heroes, and then I collapsed again.

Fortunately, that was almost certainly due to my reaction to an antibiotic. I'm not a coward, but maybe lacking courage sometimes. But, because of my faith, I was okay with the process of dying. Don't get me wrong, I'm not too keen about it. I'd love to get another 10 or 20 years because there are a lot of things I want to do. I'm prepared to die, of course; I don't have a choice.

There's so much more I want to achieve and do in my life, but from a Christian point of view, it's a win-win.

Maybe that's a selfish way of looking at it. I struggle with some parts of the Bible, including interpretations around heaven and things like that. We're getting quite spiritual here, but it's a great place. It's a utopia, so from a personal, selfish point of view, it's almost like being in heaven is the best place to be.

But from a non-selfish point of view, I want to do much more of what I feel I'm called to do. It is early days with Kintsugi Heroes, but I'm incredibly excited about where that's heading.

If possible, I'd like to see some great-grandkids, and I'll need to be around for another 10 or 15 years for that. Of course, the trend now is having no kids at all or having them later on. If my grandkids ever listen to this, 'Get on with it, guys! After marriage, of course, find the right partner!'

My mission is fuelled partly by legacy, but it's not pride with legacy. It's not, 'Oh, look what I've done.'

It's the fact this is going to continue. The ripple effect will continue and keep growing. When the new, improved Ian comes in and takes over the organisation, it will continue. I love that. It's the same with Mentoring Men. There's enormous potential.

I'm delighted to contemplate the thought of helping recreate the village through storytelling and helping people with their challenges. As I said, not from a pride point of view, but because it's helping fulfil the purpose I've been given.

I'd like to think that most people don't regret their interaction with me. It's a powerful concept when those positive interactions happen when you're not doing anything at all. You meet people and have an impact on them, and then they'll go out and have an impact on others.

One of the things we've done through Connecting Seniors is set up a community choir; it's a mixture of different situations. I turn up there and could be deceiving myself, but I feel like the choir's youngest member.

There are people there with Parkinson's and Alzheimer's in all sorts of different situations. We sing along, and I enjoy that, but I see my role there as just a participant. I want to build connections. If I see someone on their own at morning tea after the singing, I just want to go over and chat with them and support them.

Last time, a guy with a physical disability was sitting on his own. I went over and sat next to him, hearing a bit of his story, and he opened up to me. I feel that's a role for me. I don't know if I'm making that clear. There's just participation.

I'm here for me, or I'm here because I want to give back in some way based on my capabilities. Maybe down the track, I'll be there just for me.

Up until very recently, if people asked, 'Who are you?' I would define myself by my roles. I'm a father, I'm a husband, I'm a great-grandfather, I'm a friend, I'm a brother, whatever—a whole bunch of different things. Then, through Mentoring Men, I learned a lot about what it's like to be what I call a life mentor.

Sometimes, in a discussion, suddenly, I'd feel, Ian, you need to be quiet and put on your mentor hat, then continue with that. With these different roles, sometimes I envisaged putting it on, like, with this person that the choir. It was okay. Now I've just got to be. It's going to be a friendly role. But it occurred to me, that's not who Ian is.

Ian's not someone who plays all these different roles. Who is the genuine Ian? It's evolved. I hadn't really thought that much about it until recently. Maybe some people go through life never really knowing who they are, and I'm still not sure who I am.

One of the attributes is a set of values I've got, and I'm still working through that. But I tend to always come back, well, this is what I do, but I'm still trying to work out who I am.

I'm someone with a lot of empathy who cares for others. I'm someone who has Christian values, but who also says dumb thing sometimes. Someone who still has inappropriate emotions sometimes. I don't want to sugar-coat it, but sometimes I don't even like myself. So, that's the real Ian.

It's important to build connections. A couple of days ago, I listened to Dr Rob Gordon, a clinical psychologist we met through the Alpine bushfires. He talked about the importance of social capital. He said that after a traumatic event, far more important than money and infrastructure was social capital. He was talking about natural disasters and trauma. But the trauma could be a loss of a partner or a loss of a physical capability or whatever, so I think social capital is very important.

Building those connections, whether going to the community choir or getting involved in different groups. There's a lot of science around the benefits of volunteering. I encourage it around physical exercise and activities that maintain mental acuity.

I love this intergenerational thing. There are many things that older people can do in their best interest, and society could do much to facilitate that. As I said at the start, it's an untapped resource. If we understand it, there's a tremendous win-win here.

In my working career, I saw traditional retirement and not being critical as self-centred. It's playing golf three times a week, or the grey nomads or travelling around or whatever. As I said, on the 10th of September 2013, my definition of that changed. The last ten years have been the most fulfilling, enjoyable, purpose-filled time of my life, and I've learned a lot. I encourage people around those sorts of things. In giving back and volunteering, they'll get all the benefits I discussed.

One of the things I've learned I don't need now, is the materialism that we can sometimes get sucked into. For example, my car is a 2007 model, so if it still goes, it's fine.

Also, becoming more loving and less judgmental. There's huge freedom in those sorts of things. I've learned that the things that we were educated or influenced to think were important aren't really that important.

The important thing is that these social connections and relationships are making the world a better place.

My treasure is the knowledge I've gained and understanding the impact of that on making the world a better place. The treasure is this family. I'm absolutely blessed with four kids and twelve grandkids that, to be honest, I probably didn't appreciate at different times. I'm sure my kids would say I'm still not appreciating to the full degree. One of my challenges is balancing the things I feel called to do and family life. It's one of the hardest things I've got with my current situation. But the treasure of my family and of being married to Helen for 41 years—with challenges.

I would encourage older Australians to know, firstly, that they're valued and that they've got an important part to play in our society. They have so many gifts that they can give to the community. I would encourage them to look for connection opportunities, look for ways they can give back, and go and do things for other people.

Apart from my faith and exercise, something that keeps me going is partly that I'm incredibly competitive, and it could be good or bad. I don't know if that goes back to all the insecurity I had as a kid, where it was like needing to prove myself all the time. If I say I will do something, I'll put every effort into doing that. I started writing a book a while ago. I've now committed to have it done by my birthday in March next year. So, if I'm still alive, there will be a book, at least a draft, complete.

It's this persistence. I talk about ready, aim, and fire, which describe how I approach things. I meet a lot of people along the journey, and I find far more people in the Ready. Aim. Ready. Aim. Ready. I wonder if it's analysis, paralysis, or procrastination. They just struggle to fire.

That's at one extreme. The lesser extreme is fire with no plan. I'm in that middle thing, with determination and persistence. There are many stories throughout my life of that persistence. I just kept going and going and going, whether it be a physical activity or running a few different businesses. One of my strengths is persistence, which is to keep going when many others would stop.

My faith is part of that. Firstly, it's a struggle for me. There are people I meet in Christian circles who are constantly interacting with God; in some ways, I'm jealous of those people. That's not where I'm at. Most of the time, I'm in my own headspace doing the things that I feel need to be done. For me, it's important to go to church because it helps me get centred or to spend some time focused on helping me get centred.

Often, it's only when I look back that I can see a divine influence in the things that have happened to me. The faith journey has evolved and is still evolving. As I mentioned before, I'm a Christian, but I struggle with some aspects of the Bible.

It is the things said that fail the pub test. But as Mark Twain said, 'It's not the things I don't understand about the Bible that concern me, it's the things I do.'

I come back to the Apostles' Creed, that core belief I'm locked in on. I have a lot of questions about the other stuff, such as the role of women in preaching, and genocides.

I think everyone should carefully question what's going on at the moment. One of my concerns is about this polarisation driven by social media. We're conducting an experiment that's never been done before. We don't know how it's going to turn out around social media, but there are many negative signs.

I like this model where we've got a wire that almost goes to the opposite point. Yes, no, black, white, whatever, right or wrong. But it never gets there. Then there's a bead on the wire. Some people are so locked into either extreme that if you were to say to them, 'What information would you need to hear for you to change your position?' A likely response could be, 'There's nothing you can say or tell me that would change my position.' That's a very foolish attitude to have.

We're seeing that in American politics. I'm incredibly concerned and just gobsmacked by some of the things that are happening. I feel a bit distressed, and I've been praying about that situation.

But we can be positive. There are so many factors in this. My background is in IT, so changes are going on all over the place. But how do you know the impact of what you're doing? Let me explain the starfish model.

A guy is looking down on the beach. He sees someone walking along the beach, frequently bending down, picking up something and throwing it into the water. As he gets closer to the beach, you can see it littered with thousands of starfish. This person goes over to the person picking them up and asks, 'What are you doing?'

He said, 'Well, they're out in the sun. They're going to die unless they get back into the water.'

The guy said to him, 'But the beach has got thousands and thousands of them, what possible difference can you make?'

He looked at the one in his hand and said, 'Well, it's making a difference to this one.' And he threw it back in.

There are all these trends going the wrong way. For example, there are a lot of young guys without a positive male role model, all such negative stuff. But what we've seen through the podcast, through the storytelling, and through the responses we're getting is that we are making a difference.

People who share their stories talk about the therapeutic benefits. They're sharing it with someone who listens to them and hears them, and that's incredibly empowering. Then there are the people who are picking up these stories. People often think they are the only ones who feel this way; no one knows what I've gone through.

When they hear a story that resonates with them and encourages them to reach out and talk to someone else, the trend could keep going down.

We're one of the players who are doing their bit to improve the world we live in. Hopefully, that impact will get bigger and bigger. Again, I encourage other people to get involved in something like this. Find whatever it is, find your Kintsugi Heroes, find your Mentoring Men, whatever that thing is for you. Then, give it a crack and make a difference. It's worthwhile just for one starfish.

I've got two big dreams around this. The first dream is that every week in every community, a group of people get together, maybe with a facilitator, and share stories over a cup of tea. People get listened to and feel encouraged. That connection builds social capital, and it goes on every week.

Then, from the love behind the scenes of all that, the second dream is that someone going through a life challenge can readily find a resource. Whether it be a podcast, radio broadcast, book, workshop, or one of those events I just talked about, where they connect with the storyteller whose story resonates with their situation, and it gives them some hope and some inspiration.

That's where I would love to see this happen. I don't think it will happen in my lifetime, but it's starting. I would love to see that grow. What a beautiful world that would be.

When I grew up, it was a village. We were poor and never had a telephone, or a fridge.

But Mrs Ryan, three houses down, had a telephone. We would give her number, then she would come up and say, 'There's a phone call for you,' and we would go down there.

We would get our eggs from the house down on the corner. We knew the neighbours, and as kids, we would always be out on the street playing cricket or football or more risky things like Shanghais, slingshots, or crackers and doing stuff we shouldn't do. But there was that village and community. Unfortunately, we've lost that.

My journey after the 10th of September 2013, started as a Youth Mentor through the Raise program in high schools. I mentored many schools and many kids, and virtually every one of the young guys I mentored came from broken families. There was no male role model, and that's a terrible situation; it's another one of the negative trends that's happened. Let's do something about that.

On a lighter note, I've got a GSOH, which is a good sense of humour. My grandkids make me laugh. 'Granddad, you've got a hole in your hair,' one of them said.

The games I play with them, the hide-and-seek, and my son Matthew, are hilarious. In fact, people said to me, 'We thought you were funny, Ian, but Matthew leaves you for dead.' For me, it's a part of who I am.

Some of the stories we've shared make me cry, and I'm happy with that. There were stories around the floods: Leith Moonen's story, and Mick McCardle's. Sometimes, it's just happiness. My brain is often spinning. One of my daughters said, 'Dad, you're on the spectrum.' I think she's right.

I've got to force myself to get into the space where I meditate on these things, but I can get emotional with that. I have a lot of empathy, which can be good or not. In the old days, I would have seen that as a big weakness, with the old confusion over macho and what a real man is.

As a kid, my dad would take me, my brothers, and some of his mates, and we'd go camping. It was about guns and shooting things. I remember one of my dad's mates would lie on his back with a 303, a powerful rifle, and try and shoot wedge-tailed eagles out of the sky, and I just hated it.

They would go spotlighting, and I'd stay back in the tent, questioning what sort of man I was because I didn't want to kill things. Now, I'm totally happy with that. I used to think it was a weakness, but now I think, good on you, Ian. If people want to go out and shoot vermin, that's fine if that's what they're into.

Many people have influenced me. The woman who had the most significant influence on my life turned up at our church. Someone told her I was an

IT expert, which is totally wrong. She soon worked out that wasn't the case. She was writing a book aimed at highlighting and reducing sexual abuse within churches.

I ended up editing the book, and Helen and I funded its publication. That established my relationship with Marlene, who became a mentor to me. She was a theology professor, and I met with her every week. I'd make out an agenda.

She built such self-belief in me and saw things in myself that I didn't see. It was an incredibly powerful, influential relationship, and she also taught me a lot about empathy. When she got a brain tumour and died, I was really upset. I went to her funeral intending to talk because I wanted to share what this woman had done for me.

The funeral was packed. There would have been another 50 Ians there, all with stories about what this woman had done. It was just amazing; she was a leader.

One day, she was in the Anglican church, speaking at a big conference. She put two Mixmasters on stage and asked, 'What's the difference between these?' Then she answered, 'There's no difference; they're identical.'

Then she put a woman's wig on one of them. 'Now, this one's not as good as the other one.' Stories like that.

This is going to sound corny. I wrote to her once, 'Twenty things I love about Marlene.' She responded to me so that there was a bit of vulnerability. How can a man write twenty things I like about you to someone? She was a huge influence on my life.

I struggled in a relationship with my dad for a long time, and she got me to do an exercise. I forgot the question but wrote about my dad, the experience, and how we related. Then suddenly, hard stuff came up that went on. I thought he did the wrong thing. But my dad was in World War II, I think a quarter of his squadron were killed. There was no recognition of post-traumatic stress back then. It's not an excuse for wrong behaviour, but then you start to understand potential causes.

As a society, we focus so strongly on symptoms, but when we go back and try to understand what could be behind that, we are much more forgiving and understanding, and there's a powerful lesson in that.

The old Ian, pre-Mentoring Men and pre-Kintsugi Heroes, was far more judgmental. The new Ian asks what has gone on to create that sort of situation. I think that sort of attitude could also help in the seniors' environment both ways: seniors to the community and the community back to the seniors.

I didn't start Mentoring Men till 2018, when I was 64. Kintsugi Heroes began in 2022, so I was 68.

Let's get together as a community and see how we can handle this. Let's work out the roles and responsibilities, what people need and support, and all that sort of stuff.

Now, back to GSOH. I'll end with one of many stories.

We met some friends in Montana, in America, and they drove us around all these old Western sites. Wild Bill Hickok was over here or whatever. We arrived in this town and walked down the wooden sidewalks. We finished up in this little saloon.

On the menu board were Cornish pasties. When the waitress came to take the order, I asked, 'What are your Cornish pasties like?'

She said, 'Oh, yeah, they're good,' so I ordered one.

Then, when she came back after the meal to collect the plate. 'Well, what did you think about the Cornish pasties?'

I said, 'They're just like my mum used to make.'

'Wow, that is so nice of you to say that.'

I said, 'Not really. My mum was a terrible cook.'

Then, the whole restaurant cracked up because they'd listened to the conversation. For some reason, Americans love hearing Australian accents.

It's that sort of humour that builds connection as well. It's important.

JANN MCCALL

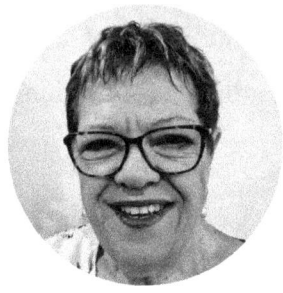

Jann McCall grew up in Russell Lea in Sydney, with a multicultural and religious background. Her upbringing shaped her outlook on life, emphasising faith, family, and adaptability amidst evolving societal changes.

Jann's practical decision to become a primary school teacher aligned with her family responsibilities. Teaching allowed her to positively impact young lives. Despite the bureaucratic changes over time, she remained committed to children's development until health issues resulted in her decision to leave teaching.

Bringing up three daughters, Jann navigated health and financial challenges. Her family's unwavering support was crucial.

Her health issues were followed by increasing mobility problems. After intense rehabilitation, she adapted to new physical limitations. Despite these, she maintained a positive outlook, emphasising resilience, community support, and longstanding friendships.

Jann's interests in travel and family history bring her joy and fulfilment. She plans trips, creates photo books, and conducts genealogy research for herself and others.

With unwavering faith in God's plans, Jann embraces life's uncertainties with optimism. She finds joy in daily interactions and contributions, believing in every individual's purposeful existence. Her positivity influences those around her, fostering hope and resilience.

I've been married for 41 years, with three grown-up daughters and one grandchild, and I live in Pennant Hills in Sydney. I'm a retired primary school teacher, which I did for many years, mainly as a substitute or casual teacher. I have many interests, primarily travel and things to do with travel, like planning trips and reading photo books. I am very interested in family history.

I grew up in Russell Lea, near Drummoyne, in the house my mother inherited from her parents. My heritage is mainly English, Irish, and Scottish, with a little bit of weird things like Turkestan and Kazakhstan thrown in. According to Ancestry, I am part Asian.

I have traced one side of my family back through jail records and other sources, but it becomes pretty obscure once it goes to the Philippines. With the other part, I've gone right back to Charlemagne. If you can believe those connections—there are sometimes bad records.

I've got a lot of crooks on one side. Now we can be proud of that; it's a badge of honour. My aunt would talk in hushed tones, as though someone was listening on the phone and say, 'I need to tell you in person; we can't talk about this.'

I had a lovely but protected childhood because I came from a very religious background. It was a strict but happy upbringing in a very multicultural community with many Italians and Greeks. Back then, it was a lovely carefree environment.

Now, I realise I was brought up in a bubble, unaware of the world, especially as it's formed today. But you must live in whatever world you're put into and adapt to that. My upbringing in church and my ongoing faith have been very important and formed who I've become, how I see the world, and how I deal with things that come my way.

The bubble probably burst when I had three daughters. Seeing what life has thrown at them, the wider family and friends, and how friends, family, and neighbourhoods change, I realise that the world is very different from the world I grew up in over sixty years ago.

What's great about teaching is that you can have input into little ones' lives and hopefully give them positive experiences of school and open up their worlds more than some get at home, where I was teaching. I was in the outer western suburbs for much of the time and in privileged areas where life was very different. I enjoyed teaching, but it was changing when I left, becoming much more bureaucratic. We were more involved in policymaking, with less energy going into teaching the children. The timing of an illness meant that I left because I didn't think I could cope with all that on top of life.

Teaching is a good career to have while you have children and to return to after you've had children. It also fits into a motherhood role. I wouldn't want to be doing it now, but I take my hat off to those who do.

Family has meant everything to me, when the children were young and especially when times became tough later in life. We all support each other. The girls are there for their sisters, family, and us, and we do a lot for them.

People criticise parents for helping their kids too much or not letting them get on with things themselves, but you never stop being a parent. If you can make their road a little easier by physically being there or helping, you do it. We're fortunate that our three girls are all in Sydney. Many people don't have their children or grandchildren nearby, which is hard for them.

There were challenges; one daughter was asthmatic from 18 months old, so she was often in the hospital for the first few years of her life, and it was an ongoing issue. Now she can manage it herself, but for a long time, we felt responsible for everything that happened to her.

Once she was old enough, she could tell people she had a peanut allergy. Then, when she was 30 months old and crawling, she put her hand on the door of a combustion heater and got burns, which we felt very guilty and upset about.

The others have had issues as they got older, like a marriage breakup more recently with one or other physical illnesses that we've had to help with financially. You do what you do to help them out and make life easier.

We pray for them a lot because sometimes things are out of your control in life, especially health or natural things that happen in the world. Life happens, and it's how you respond to it that matters. Our girls know we're always there for them if they come to us. They don't always come to us, but their sisters are there for them, so we try to encourage a good relationship between them and keep our door open.

We raised them in the church. They're not in church right now, and we keep praying for that, but they've had a good grounding, and they're very aware of our faith. They respect that and sometimes ask for prayer for themselves or their friends.

We accept their lifestyles and friends who may differ from what we wish for them or have in our circle. But we love and accept all our friends for who they are, and they appreciate and respect that.

I hope that they've learned to look outward. I would hate to think they'd go through life being selfish and only seeing things from their own perspective. I hope they gain more empathy and sympathy for people. If that's what they were doing, I'd feel like I'd failed.

But sometimes, you've got to live through certain experiences to take it on; you've got to hit rock bottom. Sometimes, they've got to live through something to realise what you said is relevant to them, rather than you being old fuddy-duddies. You can remind them of something, even in their thirties. None of us are ever too old to learn.

I'm 65 now, and we have been together since we were about 18 or 19. We knew each other well before we got married. The secret to success is a lot of compromise and forgiving. You have to give more than 50:50, more like 100:100.

My husband's very long-suffering when he said, for better or worse. I don't think he realised what he was in for. Neither did I, but he's an amazing husband. He gives and gives and really cares.

He's a good man and a good communicator. He's honest, very considerate and funny. We can talk. We're best friends and we like spending time together. He loves travelling and doing the same things as me. He promised he'd be there through everything that's happened.

People asked him, 'How will you deal with this? We don't know if we could stay with our partner if that happened,' which I thought was a strange thing to say. Maybe some people wouldn't stay.

The biggest health issue that has affected me since was in 2000 when I had a spinal stroke, which meant I couldn't walk.

It's rare—about one in two million. Something blocks the fluid in the spinal column, and if it stays blocked for a long time, you lose the ability at whatever point along your spine it happens. Mine was equivalent to my armpits or a bit lower. Everything below that stops working. If it was in your neck, you might stop breathing.

Mine was lower down, so my arms were fine, but everything below there stopped working. Then it swelled up. They took me into Emergency and did an MRI, but they couldn't see anything as the swelling was so bad. They used massive doses of steroids to try and reduce the swelling so they could see the problem. Once the swelling goes down, they saw the nerve damage. I was fortunate that much of my feelings returned, and I only had about 5% damage.

It took me about a year to learn to walk again. The steroids helped, but I had no feeling, and I couldn't walk, so I had to go to rehab. I went to the Sydney Olympics in a wheelchair in September. We didn't know what would happen. The kids were young, and the asthmatic one was in a different hospital at the same time.

We didn't really know enough about what a spinal stroke was. I was only 40, and that was the big turning point. Before then, life was normal, and we had a lovely life, and then it all went belly up.

Initially, you're in shock, especially when you're in Emergency and doctors are talking about opening you up and seeing the problem. Thank God, they decided not to open me up because I would have been a paraplegic, they said later. They said, 'We'll wait and see,' which was also risky, but they did.

I was very lucky. That night, I had a very good surgeon on duty with one of the leading neurologists for Parkinson's and motor neuron in Australia. That was also a blessing, and he's been with me ever since.

After the shock, you go numb, and then I wondered, what if I can't walk again? How can I do life with the kids and everything else? But I wasn't scared. I slept every night in the hospital for the first week when they poked me with something sharp in the bottom of my foot, and I couldn't feel it. I prayed that something good would come out of whatever was happening and that I could cope. If life was going to change, I wouldn't be one of these, 'Oh, woe is me,' people, but be a positive influence.

I may have had a little cry, but I was not down and out, and they said in rehab I was a very positive person and upbeat in my rehab.

We put everything on the back burner. The school was good with the kids. We put them into before- and after-school care, and my husband and the church were great. They gave us meals and other help. For the first five or six weeks, I was at home, resting, while hubby kept the home fires burning with everything else.

I did whatever doctors told me to do and did the rehab, and people would take me to rehab if my husband was working. I focused on getting to whatever level I ended up at because they said it would pan out, and you'd be at whatever level you ended up at. I was lucky that, in the end, I could walk.

I had a lot of support, mainly from the church. Many people prayed for me, and friends would connect or drop by, so I never felt alone. My parents and my husband's parents helped us.

That experience taught me, and I know it sounds trite, about getting on with it, doing what I could at whatever level I was at along the way while trying to go back to being a normal mum, wife, or teacher. I returned to casual teaching for a while, but I found it difficult, and I left after a while. I didn't feel I could do the job properly because you must be on your feet and physically available for the kids.

I got other part-time jobs later but refused to roll up in a ball and say, 'I can't do this; this is too hard' or whatever. I looked forward to new things like travelling because we'd never travelled overseas before. We did our first overseas trip in 2004. I got tired, and stairs caused an issue, but we've done that ever since.

As my ability to walk has deteriorated again. We do what we can, and I live each day as though it's my last. Doctors encouraged me to get out and do what I can now. Don't leave it for some dream down the track of when you retire, because you don't know what's around the corner.

You might be in control of the little things in life but not the big stuff. You've got to figure out how to live through those little hiccups and bumps in the road.

Then, in 2014, I had breast cancer. My legs started deteriorating again. Sometimes, this can happen, and the previous symptoms, like from the stroke, return or get worse. My legs don't work like they used to, so I can't walk unaided. I've got crutches, a walker, and a mobility scooter to help with my daily life. We've put a lift in the house and adapted it for long-term living, so we don't have to move in the foreseeable future.

I see those two health issues as opportunities to reevaluate my mortality. It definitely brings you back to earth. My progress has positively affected other people, such as nurses or those in rehab. Many OTs and physios were encouraged by it. The doctors and nurses see a lot of death. They don't see many people surviving and moving out of their programs. My neurologist has been seeing me for 24 years; he wouldn't see very many patients for that long.

If you bring positivity and encouragement to people who are maybe a bit scared to get up and get out there, don't hide away, don't run away from things; face them head-on. I try not to be too negative; there's enough negativity in the world.

I don't know what other roads people are taking, and I don't want to scare people because everyone's dealing with something different. I want to encourage them to be positive because I think attitude is a big thing in healing.

I've got many positive role models, mainly through the church, who are much older than me. I see them gently walking the walk towards the end. I'm encouraged that there are ways to do it and to still be positive right up to the end while living a very fruitful, productive, and positive life regardless of your age or infirmity.

I hope I can be the same way and accept that as you get older, you can't do things at the speed you used to, or there are things you can't do. I know it's frustrating, and I've got friends who say that's the biggest thing.

I got to that stage back when I had the stroke. There are things I can't do and places I cannot go. That's the biggest thing with travelling, then a trip or place is no good for me. It's about acceptance, but you can do so much more in life. It's finding joy in what you can do.

With my granddaughter, I could pick her up if I was sitting in a chair, but when she was a baby, I could never go to a crib and pick her up. Now, there are things she knows already; I'm an old lady because I've got the walker, and old ladies have walkers. I keep telling her I'm not old. I might be a senior, but I'm not old. We have conversations with her about what old means, and things like that, but she's very caring about my walker and gets it for me when she knows I need to get up.

At four years old, she's already getting used to that. She knows there are things I can't do, so she'll go to Granddad for something she knows Grandma can't do. But Grandma's great at reading her stories and playing shops with her.

There's no point getting down about things I can't do. I do what I can.

I get sad for others when they say they can't do things because I know it's easier than they think. Some people see things very negatively, and I don't know what to do about that. But I say to them, 'I've crossed that bridge a while back, and it's all doable. There's a way around everything. If you want to travel, I can help you or give you ideas on what to do.'

Falling is a big deal for people, and I've had my share over time. I've been lucky; I must have bounced, but I didn't hurt myself. But as you get older, you do fall, and that can cause many problems.

It is important not to be afraid because we don't know how long we will be around or how we will go in the end. Some people have a lovely death, others don't, and they have no say, so don't let that stop you. I could get run over by a bus in front of my house tomorrow. It'd be way more exciting to get killed in a hot air balloon or something over Egypt. The family history would be more interesting!

You can't let fear rule your life; it's about having peace. I've got peace about what we do and hope for the future because one day, I will have a perfect body with no ailments or problems. Until then, I'll deal with the hand I was dealt.

I get my hope from God because I believe that He's in control. He doesn't make things happen to me, but he lets them happen because He knows I am strong enough to deal with them. He doesn't let you go through anything you can't cope with.

It doesn't mean you'll come out of it on top, but He'll know. You'll get through it because He's given you the strength already; it's about finding it.

I believe He's ultimately in control of the whole world with all the horrors that are going on. When the time comes, He will come out on top, giving me hope for the big and little things in life.

I believe we all were created for a purpose. What would be the point of being here if we weren't here for a reason? Some people take a long time to find their purpose or why they're worthy. Everyone's worthy, and you don't have to be presidents, kings, or inventors of things.

Sometimes, it's just living a normal life, being a great mother, teacher, or nurse, or quietly encouraging people.

I know some great people who are faithful in prayer, encourage others and are very thoughtful. Others have quiet lives in the background but are there for people. Sadly, it's often not until you go to someone's funeral that you find out all the wonderful little things they were doing in the background.

Try to figure out what you're good at early and be happy to develop it; that's a gift. Often, people will tell you what your gift is, what you're good at, or things they like about you.

You know a person, if they're true, only says things they really believe. You can believe them, and you trust them. It's not a compliment. They're probably trying to encourage you to develop that thing. In your heart, you know when it's true, and you can be humble enough to acknowledge it. Maybe this is something I am good at. It's very easy to say what you're not good at. That's a long list.

What makes me happy are my children, my family, and my granddaughter, who is currently living with us. She's got a great sense of humour and is at the age where she'll ask, 'Why? Why is this? Why is that happening? What's that? What does that do?' You see her develop like a sponge, soaking everything up. She's a real bright spot.

We were caregivers for her for two days a week during COVID when her mum returned to work. We felt privileged to have that input into her life since she was young. Now they're living with us because of the marriage breakup. Most grandparents don't get to spend that much time with their grandchildren at that age. We're very grateful for this because we know it will come to an end.

I love my mobility scooter, which I got in 2016. It was the best thing because it meant that my life wasn't small anymore. We would go somewhere, and I'd sit in the car with our friends, or my husband would go for a walk somewhere, and I couldn't go unless I went in a wheelchair.

I will go in a wheelchair if I have to, but the mobility scooter was the most wonderful, positive, independent thing. I was able to take myself places and go for walks with everybody else. It's been wonderful for travelling because I can go pretty much anywhere. It's given me a lot of joy and opened doors that I thought I wouldn't ever be able to do again.

I say to elderly people, 'Get one of these. If you can steer it and sort of control the on-off, which is your hands, you'll be able to whiz around the shopping centre and go out with friends, have coffee, and that'll give you freedom that many people don't have.'

I love doing Ancestry, and I've looked it up for many people who don't have access or know how to do it. I reunited my daughter's in-laws with a brother who sadly passed away some years ago, but they found his children, so they were able to connect with unknown family.

I love connection, and church is a big connection for me. After our church service, a big group of us goes to a local coffee shop. Up to 20–30 people have coffee at a big table. I would miss seeing some of those people.

I'm also in a fortnightly Bible study group; we're like a family, which is a more intimate connection, a subgroup of the church, which is really important to us. I can say without any pride that I'm pretty good at keeping up with people, so I connect with long-time friendships from way back when we were younger.

I'm a good letter writer and Christmas card sender. Many people have told me they really appreciate that I've kept up the friendship or contact over all the years. I don't like the idea that when you move on in life, you drop all the friends who are not in your current life. For some of those people, it's important. They have told me they appreciate that I've stayed connected to them, wanting to know what's happening with them. We catch up with them physically if we can.

It takes work, but a lot of things in life do. I send many cards and little newsletters; people don't have to read them if they don't want to. The card is the important thing. 'I'm thinking of you. It's Christmas time, and you're on my mind.'

Sometimes, you don't get one from someone, and you automatically wonder what's happened? Have they passed away? Often, they've just had a busy year and haven't got around to a Christmas card.

People say, 'I'm not doing Christmas cards.'

I say, 'But the card you sent to that person might not be so important to you, but it might be important to them.' So, I keep doing it.

My next trip is coming up. Whatever the next adventure is—good, bad, or whatever—it won't be all good. That's not life. Something will happen, but, gee, life would be boring if nothing happened.

You can't say, 'I only want good things.' You've got to take everything. I always put on people's cards; *I'm looking forward to next year's adventures.* I always wish people that they will have adventures, and what they make of it is up to them.

I look forward to the unknown. I'm looking forward to my grandchild getting older and enjoying the different phases of her life and new people who might come into my life and become a friend.

JANN MCCALL

WALTER FRANKEL

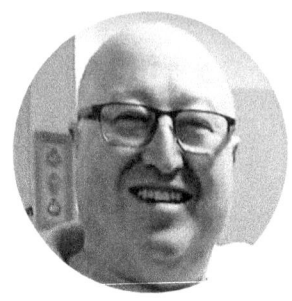

The son of Holocaust survivors, Walter Frankel grew up in Rhodesia and South Africa before moving to Australia. His parents' experiences during the war profoundly shaped his upbringing, instilling in him a strong sense of resilience and adaptability.

Coming from a dysfunctional family, Walter struggled with the impact of his parents' trauma on his own life. He experienced estrangement from his wife and children and learned to cope with breakdowns in intimate relationships through work.

Through his challenges, Walter worked to change his beliefs and value systems. He acknowledged his passive-aggressive tendencies, inherited from his father, and strived to overcome them, demonstrating a commitment to personal growth and self-improvement.

From his parents' experiences during the war to his own challenges, Walter has demonstrated a remarkable ability to adapt to change. He reflects on his transition from a working life to a position of needing help with his significant mental health challenges, including a major breakdown. This experience led him to become passionate about learning about mental health, becoming a mental health first aider and suicide prevention advocate.

He dedicates his time to volunteering for various organisations, always making himself available to help others. Walter believes in passing on valuable information, engaging in meaningful conversations, and being empathetic in today's society.

Drawing inspiration from Viktor Frankl and his book 'Man's Search for Meaning', Walter emphasises the importance of choosing what resonates and making choices in life. He highlights the significance of using life's experiences for the betterment of mankind and leaving a lasting legacy.

I describe myself as a challenging and complex individual. I am a child of Holocaust survivors born in Zimbabwe, which was Rhodesia, and I grew up there. We left when I was 16 because my parents didn't want me to serve in the Rhodesian army.

We went to Cape Town, the only place my father would go. My mother was a very wise woman. She turned to my dad and said, 'That's fine, Martin. If you want to go, we'll go. But understand that in about 20 years, South Africa will not be the same place you see it as now.' We left in 1969; in 1989, Nelson Mandela became leader.

When I was 12 in 1964 or 1965, I had a schoolteacher who went on holiday to Australia. That inspired me, so I did some research and said, 'That's where I'm going to go and live.'

From then on, I knew I was coming to Australia. I just had to find my meal ticket. In 1984, I went from South Africa as part of a team to set up a project in Brisbane called the Pick and Pay hypermarket, a massive retail organisation in South Africa.

In 1984, I got to Brisbane. The family in Melbourne, who were partners in the venture, paid for my sponsorship. Within 24 hours, they organised me a permanent residency, so I'm eternally indebted to that family.

About five years ago, I decided that I could not tolerate the dysfunctionality and toxicity of my family, and I moved out. I had a significant mental breakdown over the years. Some of it was induced by some of the psychotic drugs that doctors gave me. They don't tell you the side effects.

I had great difficulty in connecting with the medical profession, particularly psychiatrists and psychologists. Communication is the art of connection. If you are a professional, you've got to understand how to connect to the individual. It's not the individual connecting with you.

I started to learn about mental health, and what I've done goes into many pages of research, learning and reading about mental health. I'm qualified as a mental health first aider in suicide prevention. This is offered in service to people personally or in discussion groups.

I've always known about Viktor Frankl, but five years ago, during COVID-19, I bought the book and audio of *Man's Search for Meaning*. It's quite difficult reading.

As a child of Holocaust survivors, it framed all our lives. I had to read about it to find out, to understand. It took me until COVID to understand that I also have generational trauma passed down through my parents' genes for what they had to go through.

During COVID I listened to a tape that my mother did in Sydney for the university here as a survivor. I'd had that since 1992, but I never wanted to listen to it because hearing the voice is quite difficult. I realised my mother had the same nightmare dreams that I had as a child. But she never said to me they were the same. They hid things from us.

It affects you, your thinking, and how you deal with people. I think I'm a better person for what they had to endure because I have a social bent. I don't have the drive that money is everything. I'm not a narcissistic person; I'm there to help people and do things. I work to do my best, and I'm no 'yes' man to anybody.

My parents spent a life effectively on the run. They never settled. During the war, my Dutch mother was in Holland. There was a Dutch resistance couple who were ultimately her saviours through the war. Unfortunately, they did not manage to save her mother, brother, and sister, who were taken to Sobibor concentration camp. I have met the couple on numerous occasions throughout my life.

My mother spent her life on alert. My father was in the Dachau concentration camp; he was picked up on Kristallnacht. My mum used to say that Dad died in the camp. He just lived to be able to survive. He never talked about it, not a word. My mother would tell us sporadic things. For my father, it was sealed, never to be talked about.

Fortunately, they've travelled around. When my wife, my children, and I went to Australia from South Africa, my parents eventually joined my sister in Israel. That was a shock to my father's system. He couldn't stand it because he couldn't communicate; he didn't know the language. They were going to go back to South Africa, but I put a deposit down on a little unit in a retirement village here for them.

Unfortunately, Dad only lasted 18 months here before his heart gave in. Then my mum went to visit Judith, my sister; I knew then she was not coming back. She visited us a few times, but the relationship between my sister, mother, and wife wasn't great. My mum's always been on alert. You'd see her sitting on a chair and ready to run, not sitting to be comfortable.

My experiences with my family very much shaped my future. With the relationship between myself and my sister, there is absolute trust. There is no bias. There is criticism, but it's meant not in the sense of hurting somebody. We believe in each other. We were brought up to know that we were the only things that worked together in this world. We are there to support each other through to the end, to the extent that when my mother passed the will hadn't been updated it, so they had trouble processing it.

I said to her, 'Do me a favour. Give me the pieces of paper. I'll sign it all over to you; you finish it off. I don't want the money; you had the lion's share of caring for our mother.'

She finished it, then said, 'I've opened up two bank accounts, one each.' To this day, I do not know how much money she got or how she does it, but she has absolute discretion.

If she or her children need something, they get it. I will surprise her in two weeks and turn up for one of her granddaughter's weddings in Israel.

Coming to Australia and settling in was not a problem regarding my relations with my family. My problem was my family's dysfunctionality and our value system. That had a profound effect because I was brought up to believe that family is unconditional.

It wasn't the same on my wife's side. It took me 48 years to realise what damage it had done to me as a person, trying to change my belief system and my value system and allowing people to overstep my boundaries.

That caused me a lot of trauma because I didn't speak up; I let it happen. Anything to have peace and quiet, so you could say I was passive-aggressive, and I think I got that from my father.

My father taught me, particularly in his last five years, how to help people and not label them. I label a person in my head, but I don't tell them they are that because that is very hurtful and can cause more damage than good. Because negotiation is one of my strengths, so I can read and understand you, and therefore, I can expect your behaviour even before you tell me something.

My sister is the only living relative I have contact with. I don't have contact with my wife or children, and they don't have contact with each other. It is a great tragedy because that's not how I was raised and not part of my belief system. But it's beyond my control, number one. Number two, my only fear now is if one of them arrives at my front door, can I accept an apology or start again?

As my intimate relationships were breaking down, from a commercial business point of view, some fantastic people had a significant influence on helping me. I threw myself into my work because I had to make a living; keeping a job was the most important thing.

When I got to retirement, I was quite mentally ill and hospitalised. I started to see things from a different lens and saw that what I didn't like within my family were some of their attitudes and values, of which money is a big one.

I don't care about money; it is just there to provide. Yet on my side of the family, all they thought about was, 'Where's the money? Bring me some more money. I need that.' I didn't like that. I'm a quasi-capitalist; I believe in the capitalist system, but I am also at odds with various governments because I believe in helping people. But my family didn't seem to see that.

My sister's a socialist, and she lives in a kibbutz. They have tremendous problems having to deal with it because it's committees on committees who decide when things go. I'm an autocrat from that point of view.

You've got to be prepared to change. From a young age, my mother taught my sister and me about life changes, and she was very certain that, at various points, she had changed things in our lives for the better in her viewpoint, not necessarily in ours at the time.

But she acknowledged the life of change, so we grew up with that in our minds. It wasn't something we contested. Most people don't like change because it's disruptive, unpleasant, and requires giving up something.

I've always been able to adapt to change, and that's why I came to Australia. The social structure here suited my viewpoint. It wasn't the same, but it was the only place in the world that was similar and the furthest place from everywhere at the time.

I've not had many friendships throughout my life because I have trust issues, but people have always come to me from left field. But somebody always enters my life at a certain point when I'm in need and helps me, guides me or gives to me.

I don't fear because I know it will be okay. I'm reasonably educated. I know how to navigate and negotiate my way through situations and can remove myself emotionally from the negotiation and then research, find things, and think it through.

I try to give people some of that experience. Don't just stop and say, 'No, this is no good.' You've got to think differently and take a different approach to having a conversation and how you see things.

I tend to meet people who help me. My small circle of people in my life, across the world, all came to me from left field. They weren't supposed to be there, but we didn't judge each other because we had a personal connection and had those conversations. They stretched their arm out and lifted, which I do for others now. I stretch my arm out. If people want it, I'm there and don't invade their space. I leave myself side by side with them as I walk them through, and I have had to learn to listen instead of speaking.

I need to help people because people need help. Not everybody is self-sufficient, academically, or emotionally qualified to handle things, and they need support. If I can support and help you, I will do it. I won't ask you for money. All I ask is that you respect me, and I will respect you.

We may not have similar agreements regarding values or political or religious convictions, but as long as you are legal, that's okay. When you move across the line, and you go into the illegalities, I walk away. I won't get involved. I won't be pressured to deal in the grey areas.

I have one conversation at a time. I talk to anybody and everybody. I don't care who you are. I respect you as a human being and like listening to other people's stories. I've learned a terrific amount through my own experiences. What other people have told me has formed my view of this world.

At the moment, my view of this world is unbelievably blurry because I don't like what I see of man's inhumanity to man under the guise of religion and corporatisation. I find it distasteful and unnecessary. There's too much suffering at the hands of people who are very wrong in how they do things.

How I make a difference is, firstly, you must want to give back. If you don't want to give back to society, you've got the biggest problem to overcome. The only way I can give back is to use my lived experience, academic knowledge, and thirst, which has always been there.

I love information. I don't read books for storytelling purposes. I read information, and the web has been my greatest resource. I carry a disk around with me when I go anywhere.

It's got over 50,000 documents, photographs, and information on the topics that I'm thinking about. I don't just form an opinion about something because somebody said so. I'm interested, and if I believe it's worth it, I will research it.

I work with the School of Elders at the Wesley Mission. I accidentally met the person who runs it, and she said, 'What can you do for me?'

I said, 'I suppose I could run a course for you.' I came up with a name, changed it a bit, and used different words. I called it *Discussing the Elephant in the Room*. I had a whole range of topics. I changed it recently to narrow the topics but still cover the same width because I think it was overpowering with so many topics.

I like talking to people and meet them in all different ways, and they like to come and talk to me. Often, I'm there early, and somebody will sit down with me and want to know.

They may not come to the class, but they want to know, and I'm here to share.

These are mature age people who are lonely and need socialisation, and the Mission gives it to them.

The nice part is that I don't earn any money, so I'm not accountable for doing things. It's all voluntary, but people pay to hear me, and that money goes into the Mission's coffers to help them do more programs. If I had to charge for it, I would have to deal with all the difficulties people face.

You can charge for it, but don't give it to them for free. People don't necessarily respect anything that they get for free.

The power of having conversations is giving somebody a voice and the opportunity to talk about their troubles confidentially. To get some advice on how to deal with the issues that worry them, the fear of abandonment, the fear of death. What do they have to get to do? How do they talk to their family and friends about their wishes and dying wishes? What are the things they need to do?

They are very appreciative because most of them have heard things, but they don't know how to sew them together like a piece of cloth. They get confused, and as you get older, it is harder to jumble all this into a logical order. Fortunately, I still have those faculties.

The components of that space are trust, knowledge, and thinking. A few weeks ago we were discussing coercive control laws coming into effect in New South Wales. We chatted about it, and three-quarters of the way through, a mature lady, nearly 90 years old, said, 'You know what I've just realised? I lived my life with my late husband, and he had coercive control over me.'

Because most people don't actually understand the language. What do the words mean?

Now, I can't spell, but I have always been very attuned to what a word means and whether people use it in the correct context.

It is vital to create those safe spaces. You need to get the person to accept the situation they find themselves in and have a plan for dealing with it so that they don't feel vulnerable or abandoned anymore. Most mature people fear being judged, abandoned, or held ransom, so I address their real fears well.

Retirement is not nice. I find it personally challenging, so I do what I do. Your friends are no longer there; they are dying off. You must move away because of financial or family reasons. Everything in your life changes, and you're not equipped for it.

Men, in particular, find it very lonely because we don't know how to reconnect with other people. We don't know how people will help you. Where do you do it? Having the courage to do it. It's very daunting.

For me, the moment I lose my ability to have my freedom in that sense is the day I don't live any longer. Otherwise, it's like living in God's waiting room for your number to be called.

That makes me able to understand when I'm dealing with people, say, with suicidal ideation or with family matters. I see it from their eyes, not from my eyes. How do we get you to at least be able to deal with it and live with it somehow? What are your wishes?

I engage with them by just being with them. I've learned not to talk until they have talked to me. I don't make presumptions, and I listen and empathise with them. I don't sympathise with them; there's a big difference. I walk with them means I listen, I hear, and only when you allow me to talk, or ask me to talk, do I talk. The talk is the therapy of putting it out of your system, getting it out of you so that you can cope with it.

Most of us have movies in our heads, and they keep changing, and after a while, you don't know what is fact or fable.

One of the first exercises I do with people is I say, 'Please take everything you know of your life's journey and put it in writing, whether it's writing physically, digitally, like recording. Put it out there, and then take the helicopter view and start.' Only once you can reconnect to who you believe you are can you move forward and deal with the issues. Getting it out there helps you to start that journey. It may take you quite a while. I've done all that; I just started doing it. I discovered journaling. An essential part of journaling your life is never handing over that document with all the bad stuff; it's about getting it out of your system and acknowledging it.

We have real conversations about death and dying. I don't fear death personally. I don't know what is after death. We all have tales and stories told to us by various people, cultures, and religions. I don't have a fear that if there is a maker, I've got to meet the maker and make atonement because I am not necessarily happy, but I'm comfortable, and we don't know when death is going to happen.

It's one of the givens in this world. You will die, but when, where, and how remain to be seen. Giving people the feeling that they are being heard that they are prepared, that they have acknowledged their wishes, and getting people to respect them. Whether they agree with them or not is irrelevant.

It's respect and making them comfortable that, yes, it's going to happen. You know, death occurs at the most disadvantageous time in people's lives. It's called acceptance.

There's a theory called the acceptance theory. It's about people accepting where they are in their current situation and knowing what pathways they can choose to try to improve it. Many people stay in the current because that's where they're comfortable, even if it's terrible. It's because they've chosen that for whatever reason.

It's giving them the power to think, the power to choose and the right to do it. It's all about empowerment. I grew up in the age when you went to all these seminars, where you had the 'ra ra' and everything else. Everybody's going to get empowered; everybody has a system.

I quickly found out that they have systems, and they charge thousands of dollars to buy their systems, but they don't work. They don't work simply because they're not your system or your belief system. It's the guy selling it to you.

Very few people accomplish anything with those seminars. Hopefully, they make them feel better. It's amazing what people do, empowering people to be in control of themselves.

If you go back to Viktor Frankl, that was how he managed to survive the Auschwitz concentration camp, where he wrote his book, *Man's Search for Meaning*. A very similar Japanese philosophy is called Ikigai. It's about understanding these things and choosing which bits resonate with you as worthwhile. You don't have to do it all.

We should have done it at the start but none of us do because we're too busy trying to support our chosen lifestyle. We get to the mature end of our lives, with a lot of lived experience and regret. It depends on whether I take the opportunity to look at it in a positive light or with the victim's attitude.

We are definitely the only species on this Earth that has been given the ability to choose. Animals can't choose. Humans can choose either the right way or the wrong way, and that's about the best of my religious convictions.

For me, the only good thing about being here right now is giving back to other people and standing with them. If that goes, I have nothing to live for. I don't want to sit in a chair all day and do nothing or watch the gogglebox. Being able to do something and use your life's experience for the betterment of mankind is important.

Service is life for me. I volunteer for specific organisations I agree with and am on call; if you need me, I'm there. I just want to do things, and it keeps me occupied and mentally agile as I work through. I'm a solutions person. I don't create problems; I find solutions.

What inspires people to keep going is encouragement from their family and friends that they are worthy and that what they have lived is valuable to all. The problem is getting others to acknowledge you. That could be significant others or others in terms of friendship, corporate, business, or academic life.

Your family is not shouting you down or shutting you up. You could pass on a segment of something good to somebody, and in later life, they wake up and say, 'You know what, Grandad said that to me, man, he was clever.' You may not be there any longer, but they've taken it on board because they didn't judge or criticise you when you passed the information.

All human beings want is to be heard. It's difficult today, particularly on the noisy social media side, in the busy lifestyles that we have challenged ourselves to live. Having a meaningful conversation around a table doesn't really exist.

When I was growing up, every night we had dinner together, not each one getting their TV tray and then going and sitting alone. We sat around the table. Things were talked about, and Dad's business was discussed. We knew that we were trusted to be allowed that information and that we weren't to pass what we knew on to our friends or their families because industrial espionage has been around forever.

The best approach to dealing with life's challenges is to become involved to the best of your ability, capability, and willingness. To sit detached doesn't help or complain as the victim. You need to be proactive, even if it's just a little thing, and don't judge somebody else. You haven't walked in their shoes. Be empathetic.

In other words, be there in the moment because you can't necessarily do anything or fix everything. There are some wonderful people out there who volunteer and help every day. I can tell you that you feel much better in yourself when you've given than when you've taken. You're grateful when you've taken, but giving is much better than taking.

When I look towards the future, all I know is I don't want it to be worse than what it is now. But we all have dreams and aspirations. We all want to be loved and be held and all these sorts of things. Are you making yourself available now?

Making yourself available to opportunities or giving is a big challenge. The things that we've experienced sometimes hold us back.

WALTER FRANKEL

JENI VERCOE

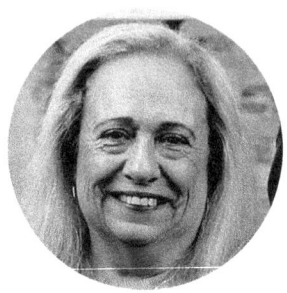

Jeni was married at twenty-two at a time when many women stayed at home after marriage.

When her marriage broke up after twenty-two years, she had zero self-esteem, two kids and no idea how to move on, as she felt she had no skills.

She tells her remarkable story with humour, honesty, and wisdom, and describes how she tackled nursing first by training as an enrolled nurse then later moving into other levels of nursing.

Her story is inspirational for anyone suffering from low self-esteem or imposter syndrome.

I had always wanted to be a nurse but was never confident or smart enough, so I never pursued it. I was a stay-at-home mum with my boys for 14 years, which was a great privilege.

When my marriage broke down, I thought nursing is all in the universities now; you've missed the boat. I'll keep looking in the paper; something will jump out at me. Because I wanted to set a good example for my boys, I wasn't going to sit on my backside and do nothing. I had to show them that when you cop a kick, you've got to pick yourself back up.

One day, there was an ad in the paper for the one-year Enrolled Nursing course, which I was oblivious to. When I looked at the criteria, I thought, 'Oh, I'm sure I could do that.'

Although I had zero self-confidence and self-esteem, I applied and got accepted. I was terrified when I thought about returning to full-time study and work as I hadn't worked for about twenty-two years.

Then, some friends with an unemployment agency stepped in. I said, 'I've got to do a numeracy and literacy test. I hate maths. What am I going to do?'

They said, 'Jeni, it'll be fine.'

Much to my amazement, I was accepted. Even when I got through the course, I remember going up to one of the lecturers at the graduation and saying, 'Who'd have thought I would be here?'

She said, 'Well, I knew you would be.'

During those twelve months, I had many tears and tantrums.

'What on Earth possessed me to think I could do this? I can't do this. It is too hard; it's affecting the kids.'

It was hard work and a big change for all of us, from always having Mum around to suddenly getting their own food.

I remember the first person I told I was going into nursing; she had been a nurse for a long time. Her reaction surprised me. Instead of encouragement, I got, 'Oh, are you mad? What on earth are you thinking?'

I was shocked because she was the only person on this journey who said that. I thought that was strange to say to someone when I was so excited about this. I thought you don't do that to people. Even if you don't agree with what they're doing or believe they will make it, you don't steal their joy. It seemed a bit harsh.

I got through that course, then I did the Community Nursing course and got the second-highest marks in New South Wales. Then I thought, do I dare? I felt like I was on one side of the river, with other things on the other, which I'd love to do.

But in the middle was this giant stepping stone that said, Registered Nurse. The only way I could get over there was to do the Registered Nurses course at the university. I don't know if I can do that, and I never thought I'd go to uni. However, I put in the application, and I was accepted.

Luckily, the university dropped the course to two years because I was already an enrolled nurse.

Then, there were another two years of tantrums, screaming at the computer, and crying. I think it's alright to have a pity party, yell, scream, kick, whatever. Get it out of your system, and then pick yourself up, dust yourself off and go, okay, I can do this.

It was hard, and I had to keep going and pushing again. We all struggled with one subject, and I said, 'I'll do extra coursework. I don't care what it is. I'll pick it up as I cannot fail this course. I've got this far; I can keep going.'

My boys were teenagers at the time and were fabulous, as were a couple of friends. Then, as I got to the end of the Registered Nurse's course, my father was diagnosed with lung cancer, which was already in other parts of his body, so he was dying.

I knew that as soon as I told him I'd achieved becoming a Registered Nurse, he'd go, and he did, about a week later. I dreaded telling him but knew he was hanging on for that news.

So once I went through that, I was accepted at the Mater Hospital in my new graduate position. Then I did my theatre course, and all these years later, I still work in operating theatres in day surgery. Then, a couple of years ago, I earned my graduate certificate in anaesthetics online.

That was also difficult; more tears and tantrums; it must just be something with me and computers. I had signed up for the grad certificate, the diploma and the Masters, but you could jump out any time after each section if you wanted to.

When I reached the end of the certificate, my youngest son said, 'That's it. No more uni for you, Mum. I can't take it anymore.'

I thoroughly agreed with him and said, 'I'm not doing that anymore.'

I am coming up to 23 years now. I got there without confidence; I hadn't realised I had disappeared completely. When my marriage broke down, I was totally lost with no identity, knowing I had to start all over again.

When we split up, a girlfriend said, 'Now we might see the old Jeni back.' I hadn't even realised that I had just disappeared.

The marriage breakdown was the catalyst for looking inside myself and saying, 'Well, not only do I need to do something for the sake of setting a good example for my kids, but I want to do something for myself.'

It was hard when your self-esteem was gone, you were made to feel dumb, and you hadn't been encouraged to do anything. So you second guess yourself all the time and don't have the confidence to think you can do it.

My ex was a very high-ranking police officer; he had university degrees, a law degree and all that sort of thing. I was just a little woman at home. He said, 'I'll give you a little bit of money every week, and that'll do for you.'

My mum wasn't very encouraging either. Dad quietly was my rock. Not having the confidence to excel in anything in childhood impacts you through life. Until you wake up, or that bell goes off in your head, you say, 'Hang on a minute, I can do this.'

The messages we had at school didn't help. Most of us left school when we were 15 or 16, and we all went to secretarial school. That was it. You'll be a secretary until you find someone to marry, and then you'll have kids; that's your role in life.

At that age, I was oblivious to that situation. I thought that's what you do. My mum had stayed home once she was pregnant with me; all the women in my life had stayed at home, so there wasn't anything different for me.

Now they've got all the choices in the world.

I had my rose-coloured glasses on, about marriage—the tall, dark, handsome husband. I was in awe of my ex and put him on a pedestal. You shouldn't do that with anybody because you're setting them up for a fall and yourself up for disappointment.

Things didn't go the way I thought they would. He was married to the job, and I was married to him. There were two lives. There was my life with the boys, and we did everything together. My ex popped in occasionally because he was on call 24/7.

Later, I realised I'd been a single parent all my life. If you're married to someone dedicated to jobs like military jobs, paramedics, or doctors, that's their life. They all miss important occasions, and you must remember that's the way it is when you sign up.

But I was twenty-one when I got engaged and twenty-two when I got married; I had no idea. My fairy tale dreams of what it would be like didn't come true.

My eldest is now thirty-six, and I remember bringing him home from the hospital, putting him in the bassinet, and just sitting there staring at him.

My ex, Glen, said, 'Oh, well, I've got to go to uni now.' Then off he went out the door.

I'm wondering, 'What if he wakes up? What do I do with him?' I had zero idea.

During the 1994 bushfires, he left me with three kids and a dog or a cat. Then, there was a message to evacuate. I had to be very organised, so many disasters were left to me.

I could handle it; I wasn't one of these people who would sit down, put their head in their hands, and go, 'Oh no, what do I do?' I could nut things out, and I got a lot of that from Dad, who was very much that person.

Two years before we split up, I lost my brother to suicide. It was a horrible time. I remember thinking then, I will never have my happiness dependent on another person because look what happens. I started to think, what would I do if Glen left? How would I cope? I felt I'd be okay.

When it happened, I wondered, 'Oh, what can I do?' Because I had no job and was dependent on him. You need time to process and nut it out and have your tears and feelings of hopelessness.

I had the kids, so I needed to be strong for them because they'd lost their dad. They'd not long lost their uncle, who they loved dearly, and then their dad walked out the door. I was dealing with their grief as well.

But I always kept them connected to their dad. I said, ring him anytime you want to. Just ring him and tell him you want to see him. So, there was no angst about the kids.

When I saw the course ad in the paper, I thought I was very daring. I thought if I go for something and get it, it's because I'm meant to get it. I suppose a part of me thought, you won't get it. Don't be ridiculous.

When I asked myself, now, what do I do? This is a new world opening up. Did you have to give yourself permission or get permission from somebody else?

Funnily enough, even when I went to do my graduate certificate, one of the doctors I worked with said, 'What are you doing that for?' And I said, 'Well, I'm one of your anaesthetic nurses. Wouldn't that be obvious? And I want to know more so I can help you more. I don't know.'

And she said, 'You should do something completely different. But you will get naysayers. I don't know whether that is jealousy on their part, or they don't think you're up to the task or what it is, but you've just got to ignore it because I believe if you want it bad enough, then it's your choice. Go and do it.' I've often told my boys, 'I'll help you as much as possible, but you must do the hard yards.'

My boys are extraordinary young men who have gone through their battles with different things, injuries, and surgeries. I could have lost either of them at any time. Now, one's a senior audio technician, and the other's a paramedic. I've never said a negative thing about what they're doing. I think not getting the encouragement myself, I encourage them.

I always saw myself as a mum. After my marriage had broken up, I helped other boys. If they had been in a fight at home, they'd end up at my place; I didn't want them sleeping in cars or parks. I would feed them. But they didn't get off scot-free. I sat them down and said, 'Okay, tell me what happened?'

I just wanted them to have a safe haven where they knew they could come to me and get food and a bed. They could stay, but I would also say, 'You need to think about what you said because that might have been a bit unfair to me.'

When my husband left and my brother passed, I was trying to keep my head above water and not drown in sorrow, anger and disbelief. I think it's not till you look back and wonder—if this hadn't happened, then that wouldn't have happened. Sometimes, it takes a little time to see the benefit of what you have been through.

The kids had different reactions. My youngest said, 'Mum, you are better than that,' because I had no self-esteem. He was vocal in his encouragement, 'Don't be a doormat. You can do that.'

His brother is gentler and says, 'Whatever you think, Mum.' That kind of thing.

And now, they'll come up and hug me and say, 'Thank you for your help.'

They like to pat me on the head, and I say, 'Don't pat your mother!'

Since I started my nursing career, I've had people say, in general conversation, 'I've got my divorce hearing coming up this week, and I don't know what I'm going to do.'

I say, 'You can do it.'

When I say I went into nursing when I was forty, they'll reply, 'Really, you can do that?' or, 'Oh, I always wanted to be a nurse. I wish I'd done that.'

And I go, 'Well, what's stopping you? I was a forty-year-old single mum, and I hadn't worked and been at home for fourteen years.'

Looking back on the journey, I think the most significant gift was finding myself and the strength I didn't know I had.

The boys and friends helped me get through the tough times. But I can make better decisions sometimes if I spend time alone, even sitting by the water. I find that if something is bothering me or I have a decision to make, if I spend some time away and sit and think without other stuff going on, I can usually come to a conclusion or feel better about something.

I've even said to the kids sometimes, if they've been troubled about something, 'Go for a walk down the beach.' It's just something about the fresh air and the water; it clears your head.

I told one of the kids the other day, 'Have you thought about meditating?'

He said, 'Don't give that crap, Mum.'

I said, 'No, it's very good.' You never know. Something might happen one day, and he might turn around and find it helpful.

Many older women were stuck in these traditional marriages and didn't know who they were. Or when a partner passes away when one has relied on the other, they're lost. They don't know what to do. I saw it with my own mother when my dad passed. She had no idea and used to go on, 'I used to be quite a capable person before your father.'

When men retire, and they've been in management roles, they take over, which drives many women up the wall. They go, 'Oh, I'm going to kill him if he doesn't…'

You have it inside you. You just have to find it.

My son hates me saying, 'What's your passion?'

He said, 'Oh Lord, what a load of rubbish.'

So I said, 'What's something you want to do?'

He said, 'I want to be a rock star, but that's never going to happen.'

I went, 'Well. You never know, just keep trying.'

If you really want to do something, you've just got to figure out how. For example, when I thought I'd missed the boat with nursing, this ad in the paper changed everything. I didn't even realise that there was a level of nursing called enrolled nurses.

You may not even realise that what you want to do, there may be another way to get into it than what you traditionally thought it was. Research it, look for it, find out, and ask questions.

If you are in that space where you don't believe in yourself, think you're not good enough or maybe are in a disempowering relationship, I say to you to trust that inner voice. Don't let someone steal your joy. That is your joy. If they're trying to steal your joy, it's because something's wrong in their heart or their life. Jealousy, or something they've missed out on somewhere along the line.

It's not your fault; that's their stuff. Let them own it and deal with it. Everyone's got their little part to play, and it's like a big puzzle. We all fit in somewhere, and you could save someone's life.

You could end up speaking to someone who is down and stop them from doing something they would regret later. Listen to that voice inside. Because even if it's just a tiny flame, fan it, and it will end up a roaring fire. Look out!

JENI VERCOE

BILL KABLE

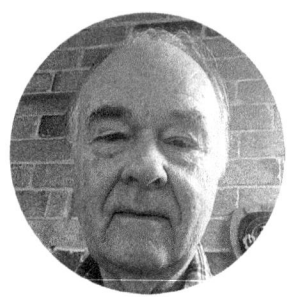

Bill Kable is a practicing lawyer who can trace his family origins back to convict settlement in Australia. His early life experiences have given him unique insights, which he's eager to share with others.

Bill is vastly experienced in telling and eliciting stories. His experience with the family courts and Child Support Agency led him to becoming a major figure in the Dads on the Air broadcasting network, which aims to support and connect fathers from all walks of life, across Australia and internationally.

I've been a practising lawyer for 50 years. But I still feel funny when you talk about seniors. I'm a fifth-generation descendant of Henry Kable, who was on the First Fleet, and he had the first marriage in Australia, and the first lawsuit in Australia.

Some people say we're still in the same line of work, being convicts and lawyers. He also had the first pub in Australia, so he was very important in the establishment of Australia. As a child, like Forrest Gump, I was there at some significant moments, like the Beatles' first concert in Australia in 1964, and the first State of Origin game in 1980.

Many years ago, when I was a student, there was a sign talking about sperm donation, so I made some donations and didn't think any more about it for years. It was an IVF program for women at a rural hospital, and I got about $20 each time I went.

About five years ago, my son, who'd come from this sperm donation, contacted me out of the blue. I chatted with him only briefly as I was going away. Then I called back, and he said, 'There's something else I better tell you. I've got a sister, and you're her father, too.' It was my past coming back and tapping me on the shoulder.

Suddenly I had two new children, and now I have three new grandchildren. My son and I get on very well. But the daughter never wanted to acknowledge how she was conceived, so I haven't had a chance to meet with her.

When I got the call, my jaw hit the floor because the first comment was, 'I don't know quite how to put this, but you're my father.' Then he said, 'I don't want to put any claim on you. I'm quite independent and in a good relationship. I just wanted to thank you for my existence.'

It was strange. Then, sometime later, when we went out to dinner, I met the mother of my child for the first time when he was 30 years old.

He invited his mother and his partner, and I brought mine, and I thought he was an exceptionally nice bloke. I was so proud of him. There was some linking, but there wasn't a great feeling of communion or anything like that. I'm sure he's the same.

Some people say he's got a Kable head, but I'm not sure. I've had two children through my marriage, and they're very different from this child, so I can't point to many family resemblances to him. I've only seen photos of my daughter, but there might be something there. It's hard to tell.

I always enjoy seeing him, but he's built his own life. I would have welcomed him into our family gatherings if he wanted to, but he hasn't done that. We've met several times, and he's met my children. Of course, there are tricky elements, and I had to tell my children about them.

There is a law in New South Wales to say that a child conceived this way cannot make a claim on your estate. They needn't have worried about losing the money under the will or anything like that. Then I had to tell my sisters, so many issues suddenly came up. The Department of Health assured me there were no more children, which was a relief.

When I made the donation, they told me a few interesting things. One was that the professor said to me, 'You might worry about unconscious incest if one of these children happened to meet one of your other children later in life.' He said, 'But needn't worry about that; we believe the husband is not the father for one in four children.' That was a bit of a shock.

They also said, 'You'll never hear from these children again.' However, there is now an opportunity in New South Wales to go on a register, and if both the father and the child consent, they can arrange a meeting.

The mother knew little about me. She knew I was a lawyer, and I think she knew I had blond hair. There was very little screening done apart from a quick question about hereditary diseases, but there was no examination or anything like that.

She took it on trust, and I think she had 17 visits before she got pregnant. Then it worked so well that she returned and said, 'I want the same father again,' so she had a second child.

Telling the children was a bit complicated as I was separated from them.

That's how I got involved with Dads on the Air because with the family court, even though there was never any accusation made against me of being a drunk, a gambler, a womaniser or anything else, they still wouldn't let me see my children. The most I ever got was four days in fourteen. I fought in the family court for seven years, trying to see those kids until I finally gave up.

My youngest child was coming up to 12. The family court loses interest in children aged about 12 or 13. I didn't see them then for 10 years after that.

But then an amazing thing happened. I was minding my own business when the phone rang. It was my son. I hadn't spoken to him for years, but he just said, 'I'm coming to Sydney. Would you like to catch up?' I jumped at that, and then my daughter followed not long after.

We managed to restore the relationship, but there will always be that 10-year gap.

The mother was an alienator, so she turned the children against me; I had some dreadful scenes with them. She encouraged my daughter to run away from home, and that was when I decided to give up because it was too frightening to go into a room in the morning, and she was gone. I didn't know where she was. My son used to scream and swear at me, so it was very rough. I just carried on through the courts to try and see the children, but the courts have no idea what they're doing.

Even now, you're not supposed to identify any people who have been in the family court, so they're very well protected from criticism. That's where Dads on the Air really started. A journalist called John Stapleton got together with a group of other disgruntled fathers and started the radio program in August 2000. John came up with the name Dads on the Air, and it was run from a community radio station in Liverpool. I met them at a conference, and they invited me to the studio. I did that in September 2009. We were all just sitting around, then they said something then said, 'Bill, you're a lawyer. What do you think?' They threw the microphone at me.

I was in the community station from September 2009 to December 2014. I started putting the show out from Fine Music FM in St. Leonards, which goes to the Community Radio Network. It's now the 10th anniversary, which is fantastic.

I'd like to think it goes out to many people. Community Radio does surveys, and they have a broad listenership. We get it out through the

Community Radio Network, which has 307 stations around Australia. It's a podcast on all the major podcast engines and goes on our website. I know some overseas people listen in. I can't really answer how many listeners we have because the only way to do that is to run a survey, and I'm not about to run a survey.

Since I took over at Fine Music with the Community Radio Network in 2009, it has expanded from dads complaining for an hour and a half to talking to all sorts of other interesting people.

Family law struggles to even be like other areas of the law. I was a corporate lawyer for most of my career. You come to expect things to be done in a certain way. But the family court is entirely different. It's like an ivory tower because, in the old days, the judges used to go from court to court, including a family court, so they had some real-life experience. Now, they're in the family court all the time, so all they hear are complaints from the parents.

It's not unusual to spend half an hour in court with barristers, solicitors, and independent children's lawyers, all arguing about whether the father should pick the child up at 9:15 or 9:30. It's a dreadful institution to have to attend. I was picked on a few times in court because I happened to be a lawyer; it certainly didn't give me any assistance in court. But it meant I briefed a barrister directly, and he was a human being, which was great because these people get very officious.

I couldn't get over the fact that if the court made an order and the mother breached it, which she invariably did, no action was taken. The only action available was if the father enforced it. That was a whole other battle. I did it once. I went to court on three serious breaches, and in the end, there was not even a tap on the wrist.

Although the court had available powers, including sending someone to jail, there was no way they would do anything. It was soul-destroying to go through that whole difficult exercise, and then, in the end, nothing happened. It's a bad area of the law and a bad court.

The current family court system dates back to 1975 when Lionel Murphy was the attorney general. He set it up on the understanding that it would be run mostly by social workers. Judges weren't supposed to wear wigs, and there was no high bench where the judge would look down at the parties. He was supposed to be on the same level as the parties, and it was all geared towards finding a solution.

Unfortunately, the lawyers got involved, and very quickly, it suddenly became a lawyer-run institution instead of a social worker institution. If I had my choice, I would go back to the original intention, which was to have it run more as a social work institution.

The family court is not bound by precedent. They say every case is different, so we'll decide for ourselves. It means you can't give much guidance because the court can do what it wants. I would definitely go back to having lawyers with less influence and social workers with more influence. I would promote mediation, so you don't have to go to court.

The two big problems are the children and the property. None of the reforms to the family law have made them any easier. The father is always starting with a handicap because there are all sorts of funny ideas about attachment and mothers. An extreme example is Japan, where only one parent can raise the child. That means Australian fathers with Japanese children and a Japanese mother have no chance of ever seeing the children. The court will not give them a hearing.

I look back on my experiences with judges and family court; they're in another world. I wanted to see the children on Father's Day one year; their mother had moved them up to Taree, and he said, 'You can see them, but only for two hours.' I don't know why. It would mean a three-hour drive up there, two hours with the kid doing who knows what, and then three hours back again and to work the next day. Unrealistic.

I've got to hand it over to a new generation coming up to take on the fight to do something about it. There's been no progress for so many years, and they keep going backwards.

Dads in Australia are getting more involved. My father was old school. He saw his role as working hard to pay the bills and not getting involved with the children, who were left to my mother. Nowadays, fathers are getting much more involved with their children. They'll often take them to preschool, school, and activities. They'll cook. They do many things that wouldn't have been an option in my father's generation.

That makes it harder if anything goes wrong in the marriage when the mother suddenly becomes the gatekeeper. She will decide how much time the father spends with the child or children.

Fathers need to have a role with their children in many different ways. I've done programs on the relationship between fathers and daughters and fathers and sons. One thing that screams out at you is how important it is, for example, for young girls to get the role model of having a father. Then, they will know much better how to be in their own relationships. But we're going the other way because there are so many more single mothers today.

A hundred years ago, divorces were rare, and even when I was growing up, they were very unusual. But now, when the kids go to school, they don't feel they're on their own.

How can Australian dads improve? Well, firstly, be careful who you marry. All these problems wouldn't arise if you had a happy marriage. People are still rushing out to get married; more people are living together now, and they may be more inclined to live together rather than get married.

They changed the law about properties, so there's not much difference if you're not married but have been in a relationship for twelve months. I think for young men, it is the dreaded child support. That was my first thought when my wife told me the marriage was over—my life suddenly changed completely.

With child support, not only will the family court take 60% to 70% of your assets, but you'll also have to find after-tax dollars to pay the wife.

They also operate in a bureaucratic netherworld. They're almost impossible to deal with. When I was there, you'd deal with someone, and they'd start understanding what was happening. Then they'd change the person so you would have a new person to deal with. Now, you can't even do that, and they don't even allow any meetings.

My experience with child support was diabolical. In my last dealings with them, they worked out that because I had a self-managed superfund, that was my money going into the super fund. There's a law that says you have to take a minimum amount out of your super fund each year, which I wasn't, and which was my own money. It wasn't money coming from somebody else.

But the court and the family child support agency said, 'No, that's income, and we're not only going to take it, but we're also going to backdate it. So, you owe us $10,000.' By then, I'd already taken them to court a few times. They had some extraordinary rulings against me, and I'd won when I went to court, but I was exhausted, so I decided to pay the $10,000 and have them out of my life. That was my last dealing. They never wrote to me and said, 'It's all over. Thanks very much.' I didn't hear from them. They're terrible, which leads to many men's suiciding.

The only good thing with the Child Support Agency is that there's a formula, and you know, from now on, I'm going to be paying this much, but you've got to stay on top of it. They do weird things in how they work out your income. They'll work it out in the way that suits them. They don't necessarily have to go with your tax return but can make their own determinations.

When you're not allowed to see your children, don't pay extra money to the mothers. Only pay what the Child Support Agency says you have to pay because if you pay more, they will say, 'You can pay more, so we'll set it at this higher level.'

There was a campaign at Dads on the Air in the early days when they had on the boss of the Child Support Agency and tried to pin him down on how many men commit suicide because of them. They would never admit it.

Dads on the Air estimated a man a day was killing himself because of the agency. They'd never own up to it, although they have the figures. It's dealing with the most important things in your life, your children, your income, and your assets; they're all gone. It's a huge problem.

Most fathers want to do the right thing by their children. They're not trying to avoid their responsibilities. It goes back to Bob Hawke saying, 'No child in Australia will ever live in poverty,' or something along those lines.

But he wasn't thinking that the government was going to do anything. He thought we would attack these fathers and get money out of them. It started off on the wrong foot and is probably worse now than ever. But the family court has clamped down on saying what's happening, so you hear a lot about deadbeat dads. It's a dreadful expression, but you never hear about the fathers trying to do the right thing who get caught up in it.

Anyone can have children, if you can have sex, you can have children. There are no real restrictions on getting married. In the church, they used to have to pronounce the marriage bans and put them up in the church. Has anyone got an objection?

Whereas now, you just go to the local registry office. We made it easy to get out of marriages, so maybe we should also make it harder to get into them. But anything like this would be resisted in the community. For the long term good of society, so that people are not losing their life savings and their children, maybe there should be something like a cooling-off period.

I'm sure many people enter marriage with no idea what's involved or even go into long-term relationships again, where after twelve months, it's much the same as being married.

One thing I would like to do is have more education for young men about unprotected sex. They might think that's for venereal disease, but that's controlled mainly by antibiotics. But they don't think they might be stuck with 18 years of child support and taking a percentage of their income. That might cool their ardour or make them more interested in preventing having children because it would change their lives.

Over the years, I have expanded Dads on the Air from fathers and difficulties with children. Although that's still the focus, the program is also about fatherhood, family and parenting, men's and boys' issues, and more. I interviewed Doctor Billy Garvey yesterday, a developmental paediatrician who has written a book called *Ten Things I Wish You Knew About Your Child's Mental Health*.

We have probably all been through two-year-old tantrums, three-year-old tantrums, and the different sorts of problems you have with teenagers. In all those areas, a little guidance would be very helpful. He's put out this book because he says you'd have months of waiting to see him.

There are several different categories now. We talk about parents. I feel very privileged to speak to some extraordinary parents. For instance, recently I spoke to Chrissy Foster, who most people would probably remember with her battles with the Catholic church and how a priest was abusing her two daughters.

One of the daughters committed suicide, and the other daughter had catastrophic injuries in a car accident. Then her husband died. Her book is called *Still Standing*. She is still standing and is inspirational with what she does. She's still a fighter for children.

Then, I interviewed Ralph and Kathy Kelly. People might remember they had a boy who was doing really well, and he was about 17 or 18; he went up to King's Cross with his new girlfriend and got King hit and died just like that. How they came to terms with that, then it got worse because their other son committed suicide about a year later. These people have extraordinary strength.

I also spoke to Brendan Watkins, who wrote a book called *Tell No One*. He found out that his mother had been a nun and his father was a priest. He didn't manage to trace his father before he died, but his mother is still alive, and he's met with her. But he had an enormous battle with the Catholic Church trying to find out his parents' story. It can be very inspirational to hear what parents will do for their children.

If I think about purpose, I see myself as very privileged that I get the opportunity to talk to all these people. They're willing to spend 27 minutes and 50 seconds, which is my allotted slot, discussing something, whereas TV and radio grabs might be 30 seconds or two minutes, and you can't get your message across in that time. People appreciate the opportunity to expand their message a bit.

I've done something like 247 interviews for the Community Radio Network. The advantage of being older is that I have the experience to draw on. I've certainly been through the fatherhood thing, the sperm donor thing, and the Beatles concert, so I'm interviewing the authors of a new book about the Beatles. It helps if you've got a bit of background to prod people in a certain direction.

I'm very impressed with young Australians. I've got two children: my daughter, who is 27, and my son, who is 31. I think our children can expect to earn more money and do more things, like travel, than we did. I don't particularly like rap and some of the music that's out there now, but my son plays in a rock band, which I can appreciate when he's playing, but it wouldn't be my first choice.

There's cause for optimism with the next generation coming through. The doctor who I interviewed yesterday said, 'If a child's having a difficult moment, rather than saying, "It's all right," it's better to say, "I'm here," and be supportive.' That's what they're really looking for. I think we're progressing.

As seniors, we have many opportunities as long as we're healthy. We can do stuff now that perhaps if you were just working all the time, you wouldn't have had that opportunity. In many ways, it's getting better, like the Beatles song.

Health has obviously got to be the number one thing, and younger people are moving away from things like smoking. Otherwise, do the regular stuff: get a bit of exercise, and don't eat sugary food all the time.

I think you should do that and keep your mind active. I see myself as very fortunate to talk to some of the world leaders in different areas, which keeps you on your toes. I've had a couple of 'terrorists' in my studio. For instance, Peter Grester, who is a convicted terrorist and can't go to places like Egypt, is a nice bloke who came to the studio, and Sean Turnell, who was in Burma for two years.

It's good to meet people. I'm lucky to do that through this radio station, but there are many other ways to meet interesting people, keep on your toes, and connect.

I see a role for senior Australians to mentor younger people. There were a couple of ABC programs about people of different ages, including teenagers. We've got to encourage that. I interviewed a woman called Ann Marie Slaughter who was an assistant to Hillary Clinton, and she says we are going to need many more carers, so many that all of us must get involved with caring. Most of us have elderly parents that we've had to look after. She encouraged it, and she's right. The big movement has to be towards more caring and getting younger people involved in caring. Lawyers are among the most threatened people with AI. Get them to do something else more useful, maybe caring.

We've talked about a few optimistic things, but some enormous threats exist. You've talked about AI. That could be a new industrial revolution. If they link quantum computers with AI, who knows where it will lead? We already have people becoming like the $6 million man. We have artificial eyes, legs, and hearing; if we keep going that way, we'll be all artificial.

I've been reading a book recently, it's called *Nuclear War*, and it's frightening. It makes you wonder about everything we do because around the world there are thousands of these nuclear bombs a thousand times bigger than Hiroshima that are on hair triggers.

If you look at the big picture, how likely is it that humanity will be around for another thousand years? I wonder about that. But in the short term, we've got lots of cause to be optimistic.

There are many green shoots and things to be excited about, and you need to encourage people to get more involved.

I imagine some older people might be a bit cranky and don't want young people talking to them, telling them what to do, or whatever. But if we persist and promote caring, that's definitely the way to go.

www.ingramcontent.com/pod-product-compliance
Lightning Source LLC
Chambersburg PA
CBHW072003290426
44109CB00018B/2119